The International Behaviour

MENTAL ILLNESS IN
CHILDHOOD

TAVISTOCK

The International Behavioural and Social Sciences Library

MENTAL HEALTH
In 8 Volumes

MENTAL ILLNESS IN CHILDHOOD

A Study of Residential Treatment

V L KAHAN

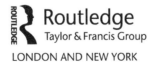

Routledge
Taylor & Francis Group

LONDON AND NEW YORK

First published in 1971 by
Tavistock Publications Limited

Published in 2001 by
Routledge
2 Park Square, Milton Park, Abingdon, Oxfordshire OX14 4RN
711 Third Avenue, New York, NY 10017

First issued in paperback 2014

Routledge is an imprint of the Taylor and Francis Group, an informa business

British Library Cataloguing in Publication Data
A CIP catalogue record for this book
is available from the British Library

Mental Illness in Childhood
ISBN 0-415-26452-9
Mental Health: 8 Volumes
ISBN 0-415-26511-8
The International Behavioural and Social Sciences Library
112 Volumes
ISBN 0-415-25670-4

ISBN 13: 978-1-138-87589-0 (pbk)
ISBN 13: 978-0-415-26452-5 (hbk)

Mental Illness in Childhood

A STUDY OF RESIDENTIAL TREATMENT

V. L. KAHAN

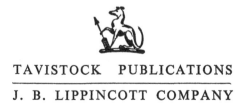

TAVISTOCK   PUBLICATIONS

J. B. LIPPINCOTT COMPANY

First published in 1971
by Tavistock Publications Limited
2 Park Square, Milton Park, Abingdon, Oxon, OX14 4RN
in 10 on 12 point Times New Roman
by Butler & Tanner Ltd
Frome and London

ISBN 0 422 73350 4

Distributed in the United States of America and in
Canada by J. B. Lippincott Company, Philadelphia and Toronto

To Barbara

Contents

Acknowledgements

I wish to acknowledge the work, goodwill, and devotion of the staff who have carried out nursing, caring, treating, and teaching at West Stowell House, and to the many voluntary groups who provided activities additional to the resources of the National Health Service. Thanks are also due to Peter Selman, my research assistant, who examined a large mass of material, and extracted and collated from it some of the information that provided the basis for this book.

Finally, it is a loving duty to thank my wife not only for continuing encouragement but for many hours spent in reading and correcting typescripts, and many other tasks connected with publication.

Introduction

Human infants have a basic need to establish satisfactory relationships from their earliest days. The first contact the baby has with his mother is through the nipple and the breast, and frustration at this point has to be overcome by both if a good primary part-object relationship is to be made. From this first step further object relationships stem. The attitude the child develops to his mother, or mother substitute, colours his ability to cope with the basic reactiveness that leads to normal development during physical growth and maturation. The process moves from oral and partial contact satisfactions to those in which the whole person is identified. The baby's successful emotional reactions depend on varying degrees of innate robustness and on whether the emotional and physical management he receives is satisfactory.

It will be seen in this book that there are many points at which either the contribution made by the child's personality or the parents' attitudes and management have played a part in the development of mental illness. Prematurity, natal stress, or adverse post-natal care are frequently found. Other children succumbed to psychic pressures during their second, third, or fourth years of life, although they suffered no recognizable physical stresses. Children who were handicapped by brain damage, retardation, physical disabilities, or poor genetic endowment, and had their manifest difficulties made worse by poor mothering, or mismanagement, also appear among the cases in this book.

The human being is highly vulnerable not only in babyhood but throughout childhood, and reacts more sharply than at later stages of development. There is no clear-cut pattern of expected behaviour or development beyond certain broad limits because of the very fluidity of the situation. Exceptionally vulnerable and mishandled children show a more extreme variety of behaviour than others, but in spite of this the line between maladjustment and mental illness is usually clear. Emotional and social maladjustment in children, as distinct from abnormality, has been the treatment sphere of child and family guidance services. They have not generally faced the pressures exerted by psychotic or severely subnormal children, with or without psychosis, and children suffering from conduct disorders that are too serious to be coped with in the ordinary home and school setting or within special educational institutions. For these cases, something more than the resources of community and education services, however sensitive or effective, is needed. Residential treatment is a fundamental part of that, and this book is a description of one attempt to provide such treatment for a number of very seriously mentally disturbed children, and of how their personal conditions were affected by the treatment received.

Case histories occupy a large place because they are essential for an understanding of the complex interplay between mental illness, treatment, environmental factors in the treatment unit and the child's home, and the maturational effects of time in the child's development. They also show the continuing influence of early experiences before the child's illness began and during its early stages, and the important roles played by parents and other responsible adults from the child's birth. The statistical tables are enriched by the case histories, which have been made as complete, but as brief, as possible. The children's names and some geographical details have been changed in the interest of preserving the anonymity of patients.

The book is based on a research study financed by the Oxford Regional Hospital Board and carried out at West Stowell House, an inpatient unit for psychotic and severely disturbed children. The period under review was 1959–1965, and 71 children were treated during that time. They were all suffering from severe emotional disturbance and included cases of psychosis, conduct disorders, and severe personality disorders combined with immaturity of general development. Many of the children had previously been treated in other units for psychotic children, and had been discharged as unresponsive. Some were cases of subnormality, among them severe subnormality, and these all suffered from serious emotional abnormality in addition. An investigation of symptom patterns revealed qualitative as well as quantitative differences between various syndromes. This suggested that the possibility of a clearer diagnosis of childhood psychosis might result from the study. In addition, the major degree to which parents can help children suffering from these conditions was observed and described. The specialized environmental care which was the essential element in treatment at West Stowell House consisted of *child-centred intensive care* and *regressed nurtural care*. Both are described in some detail, and consideration of their effects indicates that a wide range of cases other than those dealt with at West Stowell House could respond well to this type of treatment.

Some aspects of mental illness in childhood and elements in its development and treatment have also been put forward. They have included environmental factors, especially the relationship, or lack of it, between a child and his parents. The degree of mental disturbance in the psychotic cases was often so gross and so resistant to management and treatment that it was necessary to search for an hypothesis to explain the apparent lack of emotional resilience in the children concerned. This led to speculation as to how far some organic element might be playing a part, especially as there was often a symptom overlap with cases in which a known organic factor as well as a psychotic condition existed. Diagnosis was not made easier by the fact that in many cases of severe organic brain damage there was no particular evidence of psychotic personality disorder even though there might be elements of retardation, impulsiveness, perseveration, or difficulty in understanding the environment. The frequency with which these children, from babyhood, had experienced severe emotional deprivation leads to speculation on how far a lack of nurture can be replaced at a later date and with what expectation of success. It was this that underlay the development and organization of regressed nurtural care, child-centred intensive care, and attempts at frequent and long-continuing individual psychotherapy.

Although other workers had used some features of the treatment given at West Stowell House, they had usually done so for shorter periods or for selected groups, or the provision they made was less all-embracing either in terms of the child's daily life or of the involvement of parents. Keeping the patients drug-free also presented clearer behavioural patterns and responses to nurturing and caring. Observation of children treated in clear consciousness emphasized how much of their conduct was childish rather than pathological, and often explicable by normal dynamic concepts.

It seemed reasonable to look at conduct as being as much a symptom as balletic movements, grimacing, perseverative strip-waving in psychosis, or any other 'symptom'. It was therefore proper to question all management attitudes, the organization of family groups, or the adult's role in crises, such as window-breaking, an attack on another child, or faeces-smearing. Viewing the problem as one in which the child had not only additional needs arising out of the illness – or Laing's non-illness – but also continuing childish needs, the unit was organized to provide for his needs, both personal and special. This seemed appropriate not only for psychotic children but also for usually withdrawn but frequently impulsive severely subnormal psychotic patients, the emotionally disorientated subnormal children, and particularly for the emotionally deprived acting-out children with conduct disorders.

All the patients under review had damaged egos and diminished capacities to make object relationships. This may have been partly due to misfortunes during babyhood, including lack of normal mothering at the intensive, consistent, loving levels necessary during especially vulnerable periods. In addition, many of the babies seem to have been exceptionally sensitive in their reactions compared with the way most similarly mismanaged infants appear to suffer difficulties far short of autism, psychosis, or chaotic disturbance. Disturbed subnormal children appeared to be more able than psychotic children to develop relationships of a normal type when their environments were made supportive, and social demands organized to fall within their capacity. Some seem to have been less sensitive to adverse nurtural experiences or perhaps had not experienced as many. Similarly, relatively normal children showing conduct disorders, floridly acting out their anxieties, tensions, and confusion in personal and social terms, found it restorative to live in a setting that gave opportunities for primary relationships. Reliving previously unrequited infantile drives for warmth, food, human contact, and approval, month after month, enabled them to repeat primitive relationships in happier circumstances. It is the author's belief that if mentally sick children are presented with a general milieu in which nurturing is made available explicitly, as well as implicitly, and where the absence of rejection, hostility, and aggression are made equally clear, then development of previously arrested emotional drives becomes possible. Within such a general atmosphere therapeutic techniques are necessary, including uncritical, warm, on-demand mothering for the very immature, enabling them to move from part-object to object relationships.

It is easy to be pessimistic regarding the future of psychotic children, and children suffering from a combination of severe emotional disturbance and subnormality, because there are usually few signs or symptoms that give any indication of major improvement. Nevertheless, the experience of West Stowell House suggests that psychosis in which timidity, anxiety, or excessive reactivity are major elements has a fair chance of responding to the type of treatment given there. A forecast of this nature can be made as the result of observing children who have emerged from their extremely withdrawn states after protracted periods of two, sometimes three, years of apparent unresponsiveness to treatment, the forms of which are described in detail in Chapters 6, 7, and 8.

Severe mental illness in childhood is now recognized as occurring more widely than was thought to be the case. As a cause of subnormality it presents a treatment challenge to find a way of diminishing a group of mental 'defectives'. The interest in autism, juvenile schizophrenia, and the condition previously called prepsychosis has extended awareness of the wide range of mental disturbance that can exist in childhood. Conduct that at one time would have been thought of as wilful, backward, retarded, or antisocial rather than the result of illness, is being re-examined in the light of the increasing body of knowledge; cases that previously would have been relegated to disciplinary or custodial care are being differentiated, assessed, and treated. One of the difficulties in diagnosis is the close association in childhood of immaturity and emotional instability. As children grow older previous normal patterns of responses are no longer acceptable, but there are still wide areas of overlap between stages of development. Personal differences play a part, the amount of acting-out, for example, often being the reflection of temperament and circumstances. Normality, maladjustment, and psychosis can be visualized as stages of a continuum, with personality, individual vulnerability, brain abnormality, environment, and personal stresses all playing their parts.

It has long been recognized that the effects of physical and psychological stress, head injuries, brain damage and infections, and the non-satisfying of infant and childhood human needs depend greatly on the personality of the victim. Inherent vulnerability in a child, genetically poorly endowed, is likely to play its part in proneness to disturbance, and response to removal of stress, and treatment.

Recognition of mental illness in childhood is often difficult when a child is very young, especially if behaviour remains within the bounds of normal conduct and attitudes. To differentiate between apparent mental retardation resulting from mental illness, and subnormality associated with mental illness, which is less readily influenced by treatment, is even more difficult. Yet, time lost in recognizing the problem can seldom be made good, and early recognition is of paramount importance if maximum effects of treatment are to be obtained.

Symptoms of babyhood mental illness often appear as variations and exaggerations of normality. As the child grows older, however, mental illness develops into patterns such as autism, chaotic personality, juvenile schizophrenia, or hyperkinetic syndromes. These conditions are probably different ways in which closely related basic processes, occurring in children of differing personalities, and at different stages of development, are lived out. It has been considered proper in this study to view them as aspects of the overall problem of psychotic illness, using sub-divisions when a separation of conditions is possible. As previously stated, it is important to differentiate between mentally ill children with relatively undamaged intellectual endowment, and children who are mentally ill but also subnormal. There are cases where the similarities between the two conditions are striking. The behaviour of overstressed subnormal children, and disorders in children of average intelligence but vulnerable personality, may also present problems of diagnosis. Correct differentiation of the first two groups is particularly important because treatment of psychotic children is more successful when the condition is not associated with inherent severe intellectual retardation.

It is for such reasons that the children whose case material forms the basis of this study have been divided into four groups. Although any classification is to some extent arbitrary, discussion of the material is facilitated by it, and clear symptom complexes and prognostic variations between the groups can be seen. In the psychotic group, for instance, recognizably autistic children are found, as well as juvenile schizophrenic children who approximate in their behaviour to adult types of reaction. Hyperkinetic children differ from both autistic and schizophrenic children, as do the profoundly ill chaotic children. All these psychotic children vary individually in their response to treatment and maturation, and show a different pattern of symptoms and prognosis from those who are severely subnormal as well as psychotic, even allowing for organic elements in both groups. Generally, disturbed subnormal children tend to lack 'psychotic' symptoms, and children suffering from conduct disorders, although often presenting behaviour of psychotic intensity, are quickly distinguishable from the others.

From the start there were major problems in attempting a classification, due to overlapping of aetiology and symptoms, responses to treatment, management, and maturation. Nevertheless, the following grouping of conditions appeared useful:

1. Psychosis, including autism, juvenile schizophrenia, hyperkinesis, and chaotic personality without organic subnormality or severe subnormality.
2. Psychosis with severe subnormality where the psychotic condition appeared interwoven with the subnormality, whether congenital or acquired.
3. Severe emotional disturbance with subnormality, in which the problem was one of gross reactive personal social disturbance in addition to retardation.
4. Conduct disorders, which were cases of massive acting-out, usually following major psychic trauma in early life, and associated with continuing impoverished management, emotional or physical, leading to overactive, aggressive attitudes in home and neighbourhood, and exclusion from school.

Group 1 responded fairly favourably to treatment as did Groups 3 and 4. Group 2 proved intractable in the majority of cases and usually required continuing hospital care after leaving West Stowell. The results of treatment are tabulated elsewhere, and individual responses can be studied in named case histories.

Expansion of residential provision for mentally sick children is urgently needed. The unit described in this book demonstrates that it is possible to devise a system within which patients can benefit from the care of men and women who have often had no specialized training, working in adapted buildings, and at no more cost than many children's homes, hostels for maladjusted children, and other specialized establishments for the residential care and treatment of children. Contact, warmth, and individual interest in an unaggressive setting are keynotes. In such a setting the treatment of mentally

B

sick children, using dynamic psychiatric interpretation of their symptoms, becomes possible. It involves accepting the patient's 'human needs' as continuing in spite of, or as part of, his illness. The first stirrings of the illness often seemed to have been associated with a child's unrequited needs at a previous critical state of development. Ingestion, response to affection, to society, and to excretory demands, and the control and channelling of excitation were often found to be disturbed. Introjected anxiety and innate excitement have produced aggression which the child turns against himself with self-punishment, overvaluation of negativism, destructiveness, and problems of elimination. At its most severe, autistic withdrawal with self-punishment and resolute refusal to make any relationships occurs. Where the personality has become more organized, juvenile schizophrenia with breakdown of personal defences, and active or passive rejection of self and the environment at a confused derealized level may be seen. The provision of a quiet, unhostile setting is a first essential of environmental management, so that a policy of therapeutic readaptation and problem resolution can be undertaken. The reversibility of the process depends on the personality of the child, the depth of the changes, the degree of social non-learning, and the innate resilience of the sufferer, on the one hand, and the intensity, extent, and continuity of the treatment, on the other.

At West Stowell House during the period described only severe cases were admitted. Intensive methods of treatment were practised involving acceptance of regression and hostility, with manifest good will, and gradual development of control as the child became aware of the need for it.

The case histories and the book itself are based on records kept over six years, during which systematic observation, and report writing were used. Regular and frequent case-conference material was also accumulated. In addition, all patients were regularly photographed in colour for record purposes, and 8 mm. ciné colour films of conduct and symptoms were made.

Seminar-type discussions of up to two hours with the staff were a regular feature and, centred on individual patients, they produced valuable material. The writer would present cases, providing the case histories as far as they were available, from the original preadmission documents as well as later information as it became known. House-parents, regressed nurtural care therapists, senior nursing staff, and

xviii

teachers would then contribute from their experience of the patients, and management and treatment would be discussed, especially from a practical viewpoint. The houseparents' intimate knowledge put the 'consulting-room' behaviour of the patients into perspective, while specialized psychiatric knowledge gave dynamic interpretations for conduct and symptoms.

PART I

The Research Study

CHAPTER 1

The Unit at West Stowell House

The unit at West Stowell House is a small one, run on family-group lines, for 28–30 psychiatric and severely disturbed children, with a staff–patient ratio of about one to three, and costing about £17 per patient-week in 1966–7. This amount was comparable at the time to the cost of some children's homes and hostels for maladjusted children and about 50 per cent more than that of maintaining a child in a subnormality hospital.

The house itself is a large country mansion in Wiltshire, some three miles from the main hospital. Relatively few structural alterations have been made. The main building is L-shaped and consists of three storeys. In addition to this, there is a neighbouring block of buildings, formerly servants' quarters and stables, which contains the school classrooms. Outside there are extensive grounds, large areas of which are used by the children. The ground floor of the house contains an entrance hall, kitchens, staff room, nursing office, and consulting-room. Two rooms on this floor are allocated for therapeutic play groups. They are situated next to the gardens, and have windows on two sides so that even in winter the atmosphere is open and light. Two large rooms used as combined sitting- and dining-rooms for two of the three family groups complete the ground-floor accommodation. Each has dining-tables and chairs, easy chairs, and a couch large enough for houseparents to share with a number of children. Each group has its own supply of cutlery, linen, and household goods generally. There are cupboards to hold group possessions, toys, and games, and the emphasis is on each family group being independent and self-contained, so that children can feel that this is their room and their setting. Due to shortage of space the third family group uses the large entrance hall as its dining-room, screened off at meal times, but has a playroom upstairs containing toys and equipment.

On the first floor are the bedrooms for all three family groups, and a separate additional bedroom for the older girls. The bedrooms are bright, spacious, and attractively decorated. Each child has a locker in which he keeps his own toys and other possessions. A sickroom and a duty room are close together in the bedroom area. Bathrooms and toilets are allotted specifically to each group. The top floor of the house is converted into flats for the houseparents and nursing staff.

In front of the house part of the grounds, about an acre, has been fenced off to form a play area, consisting of a large open expanse of grass edged with trees, and an all-weather asphalt surface suitable for wheeled toys such as tricycles or pedal cars. There are swings, climbing frames, a slide, a see-saw, a paddling pool, and a play house. On the edge of the grass are a disused car and a big wooden boat, both of which are popular with the children. In summer the therapeutic (regressed nurtural care) groups are transferred to the gardens for much of the day, and the other children play outside when they return from school. One afternoon a week the local Pony Club bring their ponies, and give the children rides and riding lessons in this play area.

Until 1959 there were forty beds in the unit, which was organized on mental subnormality hospital lines, with the children sleeping in dormitories of five to ten beds and spending the day in occupation groups. All the children ate together in a big dining-room at small tables. Staff consisted of three, sometimes four, pairs of houseparents, but there was no allocation of children to groups. The houseparents worked and were classified as 'nursing assistants'. Hours of duty were from 7 a.m. to 8 p.m., with four days on and three days off. Staff did not take any meals with the children but had half an hour off for tea and breakfast and one hour for dinner, with ten-minute coffee breaks during the day. The houseparents had individual nursing responsibilities and dealt with keeping the unit clean and washing the children's clothes. There were no play therapists, and an occupational instructor took most of the older children in one room.

There were 40 patients, ranging in age from $3\frac{1}{2}$ to 14 years old. These included a number of subnormal children who had been transferred from the main hospital between 1956, when the unit was first opened, and 1959. Several of these patients were discharged in 1960, as relatively stable and more suitable now for care in a hospital for the subnormal. There were also some very disturbed young children, aged between 3 and 5 years old, who had been admitted in the eighteen months previous to 1959 and who constituted a rather different problem. In 1959 two long-term aims were decided from the start: first to reduce the number of patients by at least 10, and second to establish a working family-group system. As a first step towards the latter, all the younger children were grouped together and ate, slept, and played as a group as far as was practicable.

By the middle of 1960 numbers had been reduced to 34. The children took their meals in three groups, each in a separate dining-room. The younger children continued to be given special attention and treated apart from the rest, with their own bedroom and day room and with one or two staff spending most of their time with them. The working hours were also now rearranged to meet the needs of the children. Instead of four days on and three days off, the staff worked for five and a half days in each week from 7 a.m. to 9.30 a.m. and from 4.30 p.m. to 8 p.m., with a long weekend off once every three weeks and time off during the week. Two play therapists were obtained to fill the gap left during the day, and this allowed the size of the training class to be reduced. These changes allowed a further extension of the special care for the younger and more disturbed children, which later became regressed nurtural care. Regular psychotherapeutic sessions with the author were given to all children who could benefit from them, and children who were unsuitable for these were seen on a regular supervisory basis.

A major problem in organizing the unit in this way was the difficulty in obtaining suitable staff who were prepared to work the new hours arranged. At the end of 1960, to remedy this, it was decided that houseparents should be regarded not as nursing assistants but as unqualified staff nurses with meals provided. This would help in the development of family groups, as the houseparents would really share in the child's day, eating with them as well as serving meals. By June 1961 sufficient staff had become available to operate a full family-group system, with three sets of houseparents running three groups, one still containing the younger children, and the other two covering a wider range of ages and conditions. Play therapy continued with two new therapists, who were still working with the unit at the time of writing. At the beginning of 1962 a second teacher was obtained, and a small class for more advanced patients, run on the lines of a class for educationally subnormal children, was started. Contact had already been made with a local primary school, and a child suffering from a neurotic personality disorder had started there at Easter 1961. This has proved successful, and he was joined by another child suffering from a conduct disorder and a psychotic child who had responded well to treatment.

The basic pattern of staff structure has been maintained over the years, and a more detailed description of it is given in Chapter 6.

Stress was laid throughout treatment on the management of the child as a whole. His personal and emotional needs determined the approach at all times. Night and day needs governed the working hours of the staff, and all aspects of management and care were designed to satisfy these needs, often thereby cutting across conventional administrative procedures. This approach has been termed 'child-centred intensive care'.

In addition, a special approach was used with autistic and severely disturbed children who on entering the unit were incapable of forming emotional relationships. Its basis is the acceptance of the child at the emotional level on which he is operating, irrespective of chronological or mental age. The aim is to help the child to restart emotional development from the stage at which it was arrested. This was carried out in the regressed nurtural care groups. Only when a relationship had been established was it considered realistic to think in terms of developing skills, speech, and social habits.

Throughout, help rather than advice was given to parents, and they were shown that their participation was valued by the staff, and also by the author, who aimed at helping them to understand their child's condition, learn how to deal with it, and appreciate that they had the unit's practical support in trying to do so. They were helped to visit regularly and also to have their children home for holidays, in preparation for the time when they would leave West Stowell and take some part in the outside world.

CHAPTER 2

Mental Illness in Children – its Diagnosis and Treatment

The general problem of childhood psychosis has given rise to a wide range of hypothesizing, and recently interest has particularly centred on the so-called 'autistic' child. For some years this field was dominated by Kanner, who in 1943 described 11 cases of children who displayed extreme withdrawal tendencies in their first year of life. He named this condition 'early infantile autism', and saw the most important symptom as a complete disability to relate in an ordinary way to people and situations, revealed in a failure in the first instance to develop an anticipatory reflex to being picked up. The children were often thought to be feeble-minded or deaf, and their behaviour was governed by an anxiously obsessive desire for the maintenance of sameness in their environment. They often had a good relation to objects, and were fascinated by waving, spinning, and whirling pieces of ribbon and other such objects. Kanner commented on their 'strikingly intelligent physiognomy', good cognitive potentialities, and motor ability, which differentiated them from subnormal and brain-damaged children. He also noted that the children who fitted his diagnoses of 'early infantile autism' had come from highly intelligent parents, many of whom were inclined to be obsessive and intellectually preoccupied. This led him to stress psychogenic factors and especially the role of the 'refrigerator mother' who 'unthawed only long enough to conceive her child'. In later years Kanner attacked the watering-down of the diagnosis of infantile autism, saying that only one in ten children called 'autistic' in fact fitted the syndrome he described, the others being subnormal or juvenile schizophrenics.

After Kanner's article much controversy arose, especially over the concept of the 'refrigerator mother'. Despert (1949), Rank (1949), Eisenberg, and others joined him in laying the blame for the child's condition largely on the parents' handling, but in recent years the simple psychogenic explanation has been less favoured, and research into possible organic factors has predominated.

Lauretta Bender, who had been working in the field for many years, continued to talk in terms of a wider group of conditions which she referred to as 'childhood schizophrenia', stressing that the syndrome was not a clinical or aetiological entity. She argued that the conditions may often be connected with an organic immaturity of the central nervous system. Bettelheim and Ackerman have both considered psychogenic factors of a wider nature, stressing the importance of family and environmental factors. Goldfarb argues that the so-called 'organic' schizophrenic is a brain-injured child who would, theoretically, turn out to be simply mentally defective under other conditions of family life. The non-organic schizophrenic child is seen by him largely in terms of psychological and social forces operating within the family setting.

Many writers have tried to find some specific physical factors. Schain and Yanet studied 50 children supposedly fitting Kanner's descriptive criteria and showed that 42 had a history of epilepsy. However, their sample was taken from a hospital for the mentally deficient, and all the cases had been classified as 'low grade'. Also, in America, Gellner has studied mental retardation extensively and suggested that 'infantile autism' may be a special condition in which a psychotic reaction has arisen because of the parental handling of, and reaction to, a withdrawn, non-speaking child. In attempting to explain the lack of speech and poor response to certain perceptual experiences, she has suggested that in a number of cases there may be a perceptual–sensational defect of a constitutional nature, possibly damage to one of the ganglia or to an 'interoceptor' pathway.

Rimland (1965) argues for a dysfunction of the reticular system as the cause of the autistic child's perceptual difficulties, seeing his basic difficulty as an inability to use experience and to make proper use of signals received. He also suggests that the 'autistic' and 'schizophrenic' child is clearly distinguishable in terms of symptoms, age of onset, and aetiology. Hermelin and O'Connor, in a series of controlled experiments at the Maudsley Hospital, London, are producing evidence of different perceptual experience and sensory dominance in psychotic and subnormal children, and also between speaking and non-speaking psychotic children.

8

It was in an attempt to find some common ground that Creak and the working party of which she was chairman produced the much-discussed 'Nine Points' as salient elements in the condition of 'childhood schizophrenia' used as a wide term to cover psychosis in childhood, including 'autism'.

These are:

1. Gross and sustained impairment of emotional relationships
2. Apparent unawareness of own personality
3. Pathological preoccupation
4. Sustained resistance to change
5. Abnormal perceptual experience
6. Excessive anxiety
7. Speech symptoms
8. Distortion of mobility pattern
9. Islands of ability in a background of serious retardation

These points have often been used as a basis for diagnosis, with special importance attached to Points 1 and 9. However, there has been a growing awareness of the inadequacy of the Nine Points, both in their failure to cover some of the most widely accepted characteristics of the psychotic child's behaviour, and in their applicability to many children who are not psychotic. Most of the Points are general, so that a number of interpretations are possible. In applying the Points to the West Stowell House cases it was found that many children, classed as conduct disorders or subnormal with severe emotional disturbance, showed four or more of the Points, including 1 and 9, so that in some studies they would have qualified for consideration as psychotic children. Yet the behaviour pattern and symptoms of the children in these groups were in fact very different from those classed as psychotic, as will be seen in later discussion. Rutter has given an excellent critique of the Nine Points and made some attempt to remedy their deficiencies by studying a wider range of behavioural characteristics in 63 psychotic children, whom he compared with 63 controls, matched by age and intelligence quotient but variously diagnosed as subnormal, neurotic, or suffering from a conduct disorder.

Although the writer believes that the particular pattern of treatment used at West Stowell House is in some aspects unique, it has some similarities to a number of other experimental therapeutic approaches that have been reported. An example is Bettelheim's pioneering work at the Sonia Shankman Orthogenic School in Chicago. Bettelheim, however, was dealing primarily with children of above-average intelligence who showed no positive indication of brain damage. Nevertheless, the principles underlying his treatment are similar to those at West Stowell, especially in concentrating on meeting the human needs of the child. Staff live on the premises, sleep near the children, and are taught to give warmth of relationships. However, parental participation, in the form of frequent visits and home leaves, is not considered to be an integral part of treatment as it is at West Stowell House.

In England Tizard has described an experiment in residential care for mentally handicapped children in a unit run on family-care lines. The approach described is similar in many respects to that used at West Stowell, and Tizard found some responses similar to those described in this study. His findings, however, are not directly comparable. He was concerned only with relatively stable subnormal children, such as mongols, and children suffering from known syndromes accompanying subnormality. All were thought to have severe brain abnormality, and he deliberately excluded those suffering from psychosis. At West Stowell it has often been this very aspect of special need that led to the child's admission to the unit.

Other work on the treatment of severely disturbed children that is relevant includes O'Gorman's work at the Smith Hospital, Henley, England, where he has been treating a range of cases similar to those at West Stowell House. In Britain also, the Rudolf Steiner Schools, which are run largely on a non-medical basis, have led the way in providing residential care for emotionally disturbed and 'aphasic' children.

In many psychotic children there is no evidence of organic causation to account for their severe mental illness, especially at the time when it first develops. Even at a later stage, many years after onset, there may be nothing to suggest that the general withdrawal, evasion of physical contact, intense reluctance to relate, by speech or any outgoing gesture, even when accompanied by restlessness, timidity, and impulsive unpredictability, can be explained in terms of physical disease, although similar conditions may be seen in brain-damaged children. The pattern is reminiscent of normal infantile behaviour writ large. It is as if the child has arrested personality development at an infantile level, often emotionally equivalent to that of a 6-month-old. In addition, there is positive evasion and refusal to make contact. It is this, in conjunction with a history of continuing failure to develop primary relationships applied to ingestion and elimination, as well as incapacity to receive or give love, that requires an hypothesis. It is cases like these, autism, hyperkinesis, and juvenile schizophrenia, that can be seen as manifest failures in primary relationships. The family backgrounds in which they occur are often stressful, and are likely to put pressure on weakly outgoing children.

Vivid and long-continuing disappointments in human contacts experienced by these children offer a point of departure in understanding psychogenic causes, and their vulnerable personalities with poor vital drive have insufficient capacity for questing, and as a result turn inwards. Many apparently misinterpret their environment to the extent of reacting to normal events with heightened sensitivity leading to withdrawal and evasion. Goodwill gestures, smiling or an offer of a sweet, may produce a panic withdrawal, or a blank look of non-comprehension. At other times the child reacts as if hallucinated.

A physical explanation could be that the child is experiencing an abnormal percept by misinterpreting the environmental message received through undamaged eyes, ears, or skin. Message synthesis depends not only on communicated signals from the receptors but also on their receiving emotional colouring and higher brain appreciation in association with previous messages leading to final coding. A failure in this process at some stage could account for the apparent abnormal response to perceptual experience noticed in such children. There often appears to be a failure to absorb experience or to respond adequately to the environment. In such circumstances, a whole range of experience from an early age may be lost, progress towards developing outgoing questing attitudes does not occur, and manneristic and obsessive activities often take their place. Using them may be reassuring to the child, who replaces the outside world, a frightening incomprehensible place, with them.

Some recent biochemical investigations have associated psychotic symptoms with the derivatives of possible deviant adrenalin-like substances. The improvement in gross symptomatology that usually occurs at West Stowell when stress situations are prevented has been striking, especially in view of the known lessening in the output of adrenalin which normally accompanies tranquillity. This suggests that functional overactivity of the hypothalamus and pituitary gland may play a part in the condition.

From another viewpoint some aspects of psychotic behaviour may best be seen as primitive functioning. Overactivity, tasting and smelling, mouthing and feeling of surfaces, and rocking may be found in very young children, but normally they diminish with age when environmental factors are supportive to normal development. The continuation of these activities in a psychotic child in a stable environment may be indicative of maturational disharmony of brain development. It may be argued that there is a malfunctioning between the primitive brain and the later-developed higher centres with the higher centres underconnected or underactive, leading to 'reverberating circuits' within the primitive brain, and a lack of spill over into higher circuits. In this way the co-ordination and synthesis necessary for normal development of emotional and perceptual responses either fails to take place or is slowed down. The child thus does not learn to judge and control, and over a wide range of reactions his 'primitive behaviour' is nearer to that of an infant or primate, and becomes self-limiting through repetition without reaching out into new fields.

In many cases, ranging from psychosis through neurotic conditions to reactive conduct disorders, any attempts at aetiology seem to require consideration of two basic factors: first, physical vulnerability; and second, a precipitating factor in the form of psychic or physical trauma, poor environment, or parental mishandling. In the case of a conduct disorder, emotional vulnerability may be marginal, and the psychic trauma is often major or related to consistent deprivation and mishandling. With the psychotic child, it seems that the organic basis for the condition is probably more severe and that the precipitating factor may be an apparently trivial incident. This has led to the term 'micro'-psychic trauma to indicate trauma which, though slight in itself, may have profound and long-lasting effects on a very vulnerable personality. Stresses, repeated or single, that are coped with by normally resilient infants without serious damage set up inhibitor reactions in these children which are not resolved by time and corrective experiences.

Case histories of autistic and juvenile schizophrenic patients frequently reveal that as babies and infants they showed such cragginess of personality that comforting them required great efforts by parents. Such children are easily unsatisfied and they often have parents who are quickly discouraged, or made uncertain by lack of satisfactory response on the part of the child. Child and parent seem to react on each other for some time with no dramatic effect, but the child's autistic illness may be precipitated by later stress, external or internal, often of little apparent severity, as if predisposing elements were already present. Thus a 'micro'-psychic trauma, such as the birth of a sibling, brief hospitalization, or a move of house, may be the apparent beginning of the illness.

In many cases a Pavlovian concept of reinforcement, through unsatisfying or painful stimulation, leading to a state of powerful partial inhibition, presents a plausible dynamic explanation. Withdrawal, which has initially been reactive, seems to lead on to a preoccupation with self that becomes an end in itself. Even here, certain drives may remain. Curiosity, combined with a need for seeking physical contact, and a desire to achieve, continue to stimulate and complicate the child's directly withdrawn position, making interpretation of observed conduct complicated and difficult.

Purely reactive autism and juvenile schizophrenia are uncommon, especially where the conditions are severe and there is a gross degree of personality disorganization. Even where there has been physical normality in early years, non-harmonious development of physical structure or function has become manifest later, suggesting that in fact the later stage of a developing process was formerly concealed. Even in cases where there is no known abnormality, and investigation by EEG, skull X-ray, and bone-age are all normal, extreme inaccessibility and aphasia must leave the question of organic causes as 'non-proven'. Probably only in the conduct-disorder group can be found cases that could possibly be termed 'purely reactive'.

The range of cases treated at West Stowell House is so wide that it is not possible to talk in terms of a single aetiology. In many of the subnormal and severely subnormal patients, brain damage at birth, or cranial trauma or infection following birth, is known to be a factor, while in others there is a strong suggestion of hereditary factors. Among the psychotic patients and those suffering from conduct disorders, there is less evidence of an organic condition, although this seems more possible in the more seriously disturbed children. Several of the conduct-disorder cases were strongly suggestive of

c

reactive conditions in emotionally vulnerable children. The writer considers that no firm division should be drawn between psychosis and neurosis, and that even in apparently reactive conduct disorders, some of the physical factors discussed above may be relevant. Both organic elements and environmental inadequacies produce their effects, depending on innate vulnerability and degree of external stress. They give rise to a continuum of breakdown ranging from conduct disorder, usually anxiety-ridden and neurotically intense where nurture was moderately successful, to autism and schizophrenia characterized by collapse, or non-development of flexible defences. Withdrawal, refusal to accept change, misinterpretation of the environment, and an attempt at personal homeostasis by rejecting a seemingly threatening world are the children's responses. The latter position often coincides with confusional and mystifying infant experiences, especially at baby–mother level, made worse by mutual unresponsiveness.

West Stowell's therapeutic approach was to provide milieu therapy round the clock, accepting the human needs of the child at whatever level of immaturity was required, as well as providing treatment and management of his illness. This demanded a setting in which the customary rigid organization of a hospital was adapted to the concept of a child-orientated 'non-hospital'. The needs of the child with his illness, or non-illness in the Laing/Cooper emotional sense, were paramount. Emotional needs were interpreted largely in Freudian concepts regarding the stages of emotional development, and relationship therapy was used to enable the child to repeat more successfully previous inadequate experiences. An eclectic view was taken regarding personal and social development, but the child's need to cope with his ego problems was seen on Freudian lines, even in the presence of massive physical disability or retardation.

Child-centred intensive care, regressed nurtural care, and individual psychotherapy, all based interpretatively on child analytic principles, were used to provide a non-aggressive adult-controlled setting that was non-alerting and non-alarming. This enabled the patient to make confident regressions, learning to control excitement constructively, to canalize energy, and move forward emotionally in developing relationships.

CHAPTER 3

The Children and their Symptoms

Among the children admitted to West Stowell House have been some who were known to have brain damage, and many others who were suspected of having brain abnormality, but in most cases the specific nature of the damage, or weakness, was not known. For example, children later assessed as having normal sight and hearing had often been thought at one stage to be blind or deaf. There were also some cases where there was no manifest organic condition and no indication of one, and yet the extreme nature of the child's inaccessibility, his lack of speech and manneristic behaviour, suggested that his condition was unlikely to be purely reactive.

In applying the Nine Points set out in Chapter 2 (see p. 9) to the patients at West Stowell House, it was found that many of the disturbed subnormal children and those suffering from conduct disorders, in addition to the psychotic groups, came under three or more, especially if the Points were interpreted broadly as they often seemed to be. Excessive anxiety, pathological preoccupation, and sustained resistance to change occurred among them, as well as disturbed mobility patterns.

In order to clarify symptom patterns, a list was made of all the symptoms that had been noted in children before and after admission to West Stowell House, paying special attention to mannerisms and obsessions. Lists were completed for all the 71 children in the sample, and the findings in relation to diagnosis and prognosis were tabulated. A strikingly different pattern emerged for the psychotic children, especially the 'autistic' as compared with the disturbed subnormal children and those with conduct disorders, suggesting that there is use and validity in talking about 'psychotic mannerisms'. It was also found, however, that many general descriptions of behaviour such as 'overactivity', 'destructiveness', or 'temper tantrums' appeared in the case-notes of a very wide range of disturbed children.

A total of 120 symptoms appeared in the 71 cases studied. They were checked against each case, with reference to the presence or absence of the symptom on admission, on discharge, and on follow-up. The list included general descriptions of behaviour, such as impulsiveness, overactivity, and perseveration, as these occurred frequently in referral letters, and specific mannerisms, such as strip-waving, rocking, paper-tearing, and other aspects of behaviour, which are of special importance in differentiating the mentally sick from the normal child. The frequency of symptoms was also noted in each of the four diagnostic categories: the psychotic, the psychotic and severely subnormal, the disturbed subnormal, and the conduct disorders. Major differences emerged, in a number of respects, between the two psychotic groups and the other two categories. Several symptoms appeared with similar frequency in both 'psychotic' and 'psychotic and severely subnormal' groups, while occurring in no cases in the other two categories. This suggested that the division between the 'psychotic' and 'psychotic and severely subnormal' is not always a clear and distinct one.

All the children who had been diagnosed as 'autistic' within these two groups, therefore, were compared with those who had been diagnosed simply as 'psychotic' or as suffering from juvenile schizophrenia. For a limited number of symptoms, such a division seemed useful and supported the possibility of a fairly coherent syndrome. However, some of the 'autistic' children later developed in such a way as to resemble cases of childhood schizophrenia or psychosis of a chaotic type, so that an absolute division in 'autistic' and 'non-autistic' could be misleading.

It may even be advisable to think of childhood psychosis as covering a heterogeneous set of conditions rather than in terms of autism, juvenile schizophrenia, or other specific conditions until the various syndromes have been described and analysed more accurately than is at present the case.

In addition to listing all symptoms and counting their frequency in each diagnostic category, those which seemed to be the most important were selected, and their frequency in each category considered. The symptoms were also grouped together where possible so that general traits could be established and discussion of several points at once has thus been made possible. The results are presented in a series of tables.

The main concentration has thus been on symptoms that can be observed and described, rather than generalities of behaviour, which often involve interpretation and value judgements, and so are open to criticisms similar to those made regarding the Nine Points. However, in *Table 8* (p. 29) some of the most common general symptoms found in disturbed children have been set out, as these are frequently the ones described by referring agencies. Where a particular instance of a symptom is given, the name of the child concerned is placed in brackets and the reader may then consult the full case history if he wishes.

Symptoms were studied with a view to relating them to diagnosis and diagnosis, and the presence or absence of a symptom was found to be of limited value in prognosis. Although children manifesting excessive anxiety proved rather more amenable to treatment than those who were impassive and indifferent to adults, generally speaking the severity of a symptom seemed more relevant than its occurrence. However, the symptoms did clarify the problem of classification, and justified a division of emotional disturbances into broad syndromes. From the tables in this present chapter it may seem meaningful to refer to 'psychotic' symptoms, and to distinguish between the child displaying these, and a child who is a severely disturbed subnormal person, or suffering from a severe conduct disorder. Within the psychotic group, it also seems possible to separate off a group of 'autistic' children. *Tables 5* (p. 26) and *9* (p. 32) ('Sensory Experience' and 'Manneristic Activities'), combined with the basic symptoms of 'passivity' and indifference to adults, demonstrate the marked difference between the 'autistic' and other psychotic children in the sample. Likewise, the entry 'Excessive Anxiety' in *Table 1* ('General Symptoms') (p. 19), together with *Table 8* ('Obsessional Behaviour', p. 29), highlights the psychotic child whose condition is not essentially autistic but resembles a childhood schizophrenia or is similar to the 'pseudoneurotic' syndrome described by Bender.

Differences between the 'psychotic' and the 'psychotic and severely subnormal' were not major in terms of symptoms displayed. The psychotic children showed more excessive anxiety with obsessional questioning, toilet fears, and overdependence, while the psychotic and severely subnormal were more frequently found to smear their faeces and attack other children by biting. They were also clumsier in their motor action. Smelling, feeling, and mouthing, on the other

17

hand, were common among the psychotic children, who showed a greater interest and application in all activities and more apparent 'islets of ability'. The psychotic and severely subnormal child appeared to be suffering from an additional handicap, which limited his potential, so that a lessening of the psychotic element in his condition would still leave him on a very low level of operation.[1]

The number of children involved in this study is small, 71 in total, and statistical validity cannot therefore be claimed for calculated percentages, or comments, based on the tables that follow in this and subsequent chapters. Nevertheless, there are certain findings that appear to have some significance, even in such a small group. It will be seen, for instance, that 11 out of 36 cases later diagnosed as 'psychotic' or 'psychotic and severely subnormal', showed passivity and withdrawal during their first year of life, compared with only 2 out of 35 cases of disturbed subnormal children and those who later developed conduct disorders. Similarly, a lack of response to adults predominated in the same two groups (i.e. the psychotic and the psychotic and severely subnormal) with an added differentiation that the purely psychotic showed this nearly twice as often as the doubly handicapped, psychotic and severely subnormal. Overactivity was also over three times more common, and head-banging more than twice as frequent among the psychotic as compared with the severely subnormal psychotic infant. These differences are much greater than those revealed in walking, toilet-control, and speech. Speech difficulties are very much less common or severe among patients exhibiting behaviour disorders than in the other three groups.

GENERAL SYMPTOMS (*Table I*)

Most of the general symptoms listed in *Table 1* occurred with similar frequency in all four diagnostic categories. In the conduct-disorder category symptoms tended to be less severe and persistent, but on admission it was sometimes found difficult to distinguish with any certainty between a reactive condition in a dull child and an emotional disturbance in a brain-damaged subnormal child, or in an overactive aggressive psychotic one, although after careful observation major differences emerged, as will be shown in the rest of this section.

[1] Recognition of the existence of severe subnormality in certain psychotic children is important to counteract excessive optimism regarding their potential.

Excessive anxiety (symptom 6) was found in all categories, but was especially common in the psychotic child who was thought not to be suffering from a global subnormality. Resistance to change (symptom 7) was found mainly in the two psychotic groups. It was often one of the most striking of the general attitudes shown, and with one boy (Guy: Case History 9) was so extreme that he refused to leave West Stowell for a holiday, and had become aggressive and

TABLE 1 GENERAL SYMPTOMS

		Psychotic		Psychotic and severely subnormal		Disturbed subnormal		Conduct disorder	
	Total cases in category	21		15		17		18	
		N	%	N	%	N	%	N	%
1	Overactivity	18	86	13	86	15	88	10	55
2	Aggressiveness	13	62	11	73	9	53	14	77
3	Impulsiveness	7	33	6	40	6	35	4	22
4	Unpredictability	7	33	4	27	3	18	3	17
5	Temper tantrums	11	53	9	60	9	53	12	66
6	Excessive anxiety	15	71	6	40	6	35	3	17
7	Resistance to change	7	33	3	20	1	6	1	5·7
8	Indifference to adults	12	57	11	73	3	18	2	11·4
9	Passivity	6	29	7	46	7	41	1	5·7
10	Overdependence	8	38	2	13	5	33	4	22

destructive following a change in routine to a different breakfast cereal.

Indifference to adults (symptom 8) was also found more frequently amongst the psychotic children, and especially among those in *the two categories* who had been diagnosed as 'autistic'. For these children this was in some ways the defining symptom, being present in all cases at some stage, and leading to the use of the adjective 'autistic'. In several children it was combined with passivity (symptom 9) to such an extent as to amount to virtual inaccessibility. It was noticed that this was often only a stage in the development of the condition and might give way to overactive and negativistic behaviour, with a persisting indifference to adults and lack of contact with the environment in general. In such cases the prognosis was poor, unless some contact could be established.

Eighteen of the 71 children in the study were considered to have made no significant progress, and of these 14 had been described as 'indifferent to adults', with 10 also showing marked passivity. Where there was progress it was largely seen, at least in initial stages, in terms of improved contact with, and interest in, adults, who became more than cuddling machines, or objects providing food for the child.

It became clear in the early stages of the study that there was a need for far more detailed observation and recording of symptoms if the various syndromes were to be differentiated. The behaviour of the subnormal child, the child with a conduct disorder, and the autistic child became clear and unmistakable in the unit, yet often the same adjectives had been applied to each child in the reports made before admission.

MOTOR ABNORMALITIES (*Table 2*)

Some degree of overactivity was to be found in the majority of the children at some stage. This varied from hyperkinetic behaviour, which could possibly have had an organic basis, to extreme restlessness associated with gross anxiety and shorter bouts of overactive and destructive behaviour which seemed of less relevance. However, in addition to this the motor action of some of the children showed unusual variations, which are worthy of note.

Clumsiness (symptom 1) includes a wide-based, staggering gait that was noted in several children, as well as poor general co-ordination of movement. The symptom was more common amongst the 'psychotic and severely subnormal' and the 'disturbed subnormal' cases. It was often found in patients with known or suspected brain damage.

Balletic movements and spinning (symptoms 2 and 3) were both found more frequently among the cases in the two psychotic categories (examples are Arnold and Christopher: Case Histories 2 and 5). Balletic movements were usually suggestive of exceptionally controlled and agile motor action, and seemed to afford pleasure to the child, but often there appeared to be a compulsive element.

One child spun round while waving a strip of ribbon and emitting barking noises, and would get up from the table during a meal, if reprimanded or upset, and spin round before seating himself again.

Jumping and climbing (symptoms 5 and 6) are considered as symptoms only where they feature, in various forms, as a major part of the child's general motor activity. Mentally ill children, like normal children, may enjoy climbing trees and climbing frames, or jumping off swings and branches, but they will also clamber over adults as if they were inanimate objects and climb on to mantelpieces or

TABLE 2 MOTOR ABNORMALITIES

	Psychotic		Psychotic and severely subnormal		Disturbed subnormal		Conduct disorder	
Total cases in category	21		15		17		18	
	N	%	N	%	N	%	N	%
1 Clumsiness	3	14	9	60	8	49	3	17
2 Balletic movements	3	14	2	13	1	6	0	0
3 Spinning	4	19	2	13	1	6	0	0
4 Posturing	2	9	2	13	1	6	0	0
5 Jumping	6	29	3	20	0	0	0	0
6 Climbing	6	29	3	20	2	12	0	0
7 Running away	7	33	5	33	4	24	4	23
8 Rocking	6	29	3	20	3	18	2	11·5

cupboards or other inappropriate furniture. For one or two children early contact with adults has come from jumping off tables on to them. Others have been known to leap around the room with apparent satisfaction at the sensation of landing heavily (for instance, Geoffrey: Case History 7).

Running away (symptom 7) includes both the planned escape typical of a conduct disorder, and the compulsive breaking-away from an adult which was found in several psychotic children. Often the basic aim was similar (i.e. to produce a reaction in adults), but the second condition was more serious, as it has led to accidents and was usually found to be impulsive and unpredictable.

Rocking (symptom 8) is in many ways better viewed as a form of

21

obsessional behaviour, other examples of which are discussed later. The action is fairly common in infancy and has been frequently noted in institutionalized children. In this respect it seems to be a self-comforting activity, akin perhaps to thumbsucking. In the cases studied here this habit has persisted beyond babyhood and into older childhood, and, especially in the psychotic children, was often a dominant characteristic, taking up a large amount of the child's time to the exclusion of other activities. One boy (Neville: Case History 11) who was 12½ years old at the time of writing, and attended the local village school, still rocked steadily on his feet whenever he was alone or slightly nervous. Another younger child (Arnold: Case History 2) sat cross-legged, his hands under his thighs, and rocked sideways. When his parents took him for a car ride he sat in the back of the car rocking, even though showing interest in the countryside. Unless his interests were constantly stimulated, he would spend hours contentedly pursuing this activity apparently oblivious to all around him, though in fact observing so carefully that a sharp glance from a member of staff, as an indication to him to stop rocking, would often gain a response.

TOILET PATTERNS (*Table 3*)

As would be expected in any group of emotionally disturbed children, a breakdown of toilet control was frequently a part of their condition. In *Table 3* only persistent enuresis and encopresis after the age of 4 are taken into account (i.e. continuing for over a month, or for a shorter period if the wetting and soiling is continuous). Transient wetting had occurred in almost all the children, especially on admission.

Enuresis and encopresis (symptoms 1 and 2) were common in each category, but smearing and eating faeces (symptoms 4 and 5) occurred most in the psychotic children and the psychotic and severely subnormal, and was noted to be related to a bad prognosis, especially where it was persistent. It seemed to mark a fundamental failure in the beginnings of socialization processes.

Toilet fears and obsessions (symptoms 6 and 7) were confined to the psychotic children. These varied in intensity, from an exaggerated concern about going to the toilet, to a refusal to use a pot or WC. One boy (Glyn: Case History 8) persistently asked whether he could be 'flushed down the toilet' or 'have tea there', and whether he could 'eat numbers'. The same boy would only use a small WC designed for the young children. Another patient would for a time only defecate on to a newspaper.

TABLE 3 TOILET PATTERNS

	Psychotic		Psychotic and severely subnormal		Disturbed subnormal		Conduct disorder	
Total cases in	21		15		17		18	
category	N	%	N	%	N	%	N	%
1 Enuresis	17	81	10	66	11	65	11	61
2 Encopresis	15	71	10	66	10	59	7	39
3 Resistance to toileting	3	14	4	26	1	6	3	16
4 Smearing faeces	4	19	4	26	2	12	1	5
5 Eating faeces	1	5	4	26	1	6	0	0
6 Toilet fears	3	14	0	0	0	0	0	0
7 Toilet obsessions	4	19	0	0	0	0	0	0

SPEECH (*Table 4, p. 24*)

Speech retardation (symptom 1) covers all aspects of speech abnormality, including the absence or loss of speech and severe limitation or very late and imperfect development of speech. Twenty of the children had developed no recognizable speech by May 1966, but 3 or 4 seemed likely to develop some limited speech over the next few years. Many others could use only a few phrases, or showed a persistent speech limitation in the form of echolalia or an inability to use sentences. The generally late development of speech is a common finding, and it has often been suggested that 'no speech by five' means a bad prognosis. This has been generally, but not entirely, borne out by the West Stowell study where later development of speech occurred in some cases. Speech development is often used as a major criterion for progress, leaving other advances in a secondary position. It is unlikely that a child who has developed no speech by 5 years of age will later develop full use of language inasmuch as such children will have adjusted to doing without speech. In addition, some may have an organic inability to achieve speech of a normal sort. We have found, however, that children with no speech have made considerable improvement in other aspects of personal and social development.

Echolalia was found frequently in the two psychotic groups, and especially in children described at some stage as 'autistic'. In several cases it was the first speech they used, and it developed later into normal or near-normal speech. To this extent it was a good sign, being the beginning of speech in a previously mute child. In some

TABLE 4 SPEECH

		Psychotic		Psychotic and severely subnormal		Disturbed subnormal		Conduct disorder	
Total cases in category		21		15		17		18	
		N	%	N	%	N	%	N	%
1	Speech retardation	15	71	15	100	16	94	7	39
2	No speech by 5	9	43	8	53	5	29	1	5·7
3	Echolalia	6	29	5	33	1	6	1	5·7
4	Singing to self	9	43	2	13	4	24	1	5·7
5	Shrieking, screaming	14	67	10	66	7	41	6	33

children, however, the echolalia persisted, and became a most notable feature of speech even when vocabulary had expanded and verbal communication was fair. It was in such cases that pronominal reversal (i.e. 'I', 'you', 'he' reversals), which many see as an aspect of echolalia, was most striking.

One outstanding example of a persisting echolalia was in an autistic child (Roger: Case History 15) who developed speech after the age of 5. From 3 years old he had been humming and half-singing nursery rhymes. Eventually this gave way to the direct repetition of single words and later of phrases. If someone said 'Have a sweet', he would take one, repeating 'Have a sweet'. By the time he was 8 years old he would respond with an occasional 'Yes' or 'No' instead

24

of repeating the question and address people by name, but his talk was essentially indirect. 'Who's going home' meant 'I'm going home'. 'Had your fish and chips?' was used to tell someone that it was fish and chips for dinner.

Another boy (Denis: Case History 6) always referred to himself by name in the third person: 'Denis is dead', 'Denis is cold'. This was common as a stage in several of the children. In some psychotic and severely subnormal children a single word or phrase was all that developed, but this might be used persistently. One boy called everything 'train', and after three years in the unit had extended his speech only to 'Here comes the puffer train'.

Where psychotic children had developed relatively good speech, content and manner of delivery often remained inappropriate. Among cases of juvenile schizophrenia, ritual questioning was common and this might take a bizarre form and be used to the exclusion of normal statements or requests. One autistic boy had a wide vocabulary and eagerly extended it, asking for exact definitions of words, but his speech remained unnatural and flat, partly due to limitations of a personality that could not cope with humour, or shades of meaning expressed by tone of voice.

SENSORY EXPERIENCE (*Table 5, p. 26*)

This term has been used to cover symptoms included in one of the Nine Points, i.e. a 'normal perceptual experience'. The interest here lay mainly in the persistent continuance of smelling, mouthing, and touching beyond the normal infantile period, but ear and eye covering has also been included since they seem possibly indicative of a desire to cut out experiences. An apparent failure to react to sounds has led at some stage of a child's development to a belief that the child might be deaf. This problem persisted in some cases and varied in others at West Stowell.

The first four symptoms in *Table 5* were found most frequently in children who had been diagnosed as 'autistic', and most of those so described had shown at least one of the three. The symptoms tended to disappear as the child responded to treatment. Where they persisted it was often in conjunction with other infantile behaviour, such as persistent enuresis and smearing of faeces. With some children the symptoms were manifested in all aspects of their behaviour. One boy (Roger: Case History 15) would approach an adult by smelling him or her, before making any attempt at verbal communication. The same boy had to be taught his letters largely by a tactile approach, using shaped letters or sand-paper outlines.

Major perceptual abnormalities such as hallucinations, delusions, or ideas of reference have not been included in the table. These

TABLE 5 SENSORY EXPERIENCE

		Psychotic		Psychotic and severely subnormal		Disturbed subnormal		Conduct disorder	
Total cases in category		21		15		17		18	
		N	%	N	%	N	%	N	%
1	Tasting; mouthing	9	43	3	20	1	6	0	0
2	Smelling	8	38	0	0	0	0	0	0
3	Feeling	6	29	3	20	3	18	0	0
4	Surface-tapping	3	15	1	6·6	0	0	0	0
5	Ear–eye covering	3	15	0	0	0	0	0	0
6	At some time thought deaf	6	29	2	13	4	24	1	5·7

were rare, and where they apparently occurred often little more could be said other than that the child acted as if hallucinated. Only in two children was there any certainty of definite hallucination. One of these wandered about the unit answering voices. The other seemed to respond to visual images, which he would hit out against. Neither could talk about them, the first due to an inability to formulate his feelings, and the second because he was a non-talker.

AGGRESSIVE AND DESTRUCTIVE BEHAVIOUR *(Table 6)*

Aggressiveness was shown by many children both towards staff and other children. At times it was serious, especially when the patient appeared to be temporarily unaware of what he was doing. At such times he could inflict considerable harm, especially by biting. Hair-pulling, too, was violent in one or two psychotic patients, who had to be supervised carefully on admission lest they harm younger children. Aggressive bouts in psychotic children tended to be more serious and dangerous than in patients in the other groups, because of their unpredictability and apparent total lack of self-control. With most conduct disorders the aggression was planned and directed although one brain-damaged child would lose control if there was any retaliation. In one or two psychotic patients, severe bouts of aggression, involving injury to staff, had been known to last a few minutes, after which the child was relaxed and unconcerned.

In some cases object-smashing was persistent and determined for

TABLE 6 AGGRESSIVE AND DESTRUCTIVE BEHAVIOUR

		Psychotic		Psychotic and severely subnormal		Disturbed subnormal		Conduct disorder	
Total cases in		21		15		17		18	
category		N	%	N	%	N	%	N	%
1	Biting	2	10	8	53	2	12	4	22
2	Spitting	3	15	2	13	0	0	2	11·4
3	Hair-pulling	2	10	2	13	1	6	1	5·7
4	Object-smashing	7	33	7	46	3	18	5	27
5	Dismantling	1	5	3	20	1	6	0	0
6	Bed-stripping	2	10	2	13	0	0	0	0
7	Clothes-tearing	6	29	6	40	1	6	1	5·7

a period, involving the regular breaking of toys, windows, and crockery, but more often it was closely related to a low threshold of tolerance, and was associated with temporary anger following frustration of some desire. Clothes-tearing and bed-stripping were found mainly in the two psychotic groups. In a few cases this became a very serious problem and special clothes had to be designed to prevent continuous destruction. The children who did this were usually psychotic and highly disturbed over a wide field, and the extreme symptoms tended to appear only for relatively short periods of high disturbance when they were often accompanied by soiling, smearing, and aggressiveness.

SELF-PUNISHMENT (*Table 7*)

Four specific aspects of apparent self-punishment have been studied: skin-picking, head-banging, wrist-biting, and face-slapping and punching taken together. Often they occur in different combinations in the same child. Head-banging had occurred in early childhood in some cases and disappeared at a relatively early age. Skin-picking was at times so extreme that it could be seen as a form of self-punishment. One boy (Guy: Case History 9) picked a large sore around his mouth when agitated, and another picked and poked at the corner of his eyes when upset. Yet at other times these same

TABLE 7 SELF-PUNISHMENT

	Psychotic		Psychotic and severely subnormal		Disturbed subnormal		Conduct disorder	
Total cases in category	21		15		17		18	
	N	%	N	%	N	%	N	%
1 Skin-picking	4	19	1	6·6	0	0	1	5·7
2 Head-banging	6	29	3	20	2	12	2	11·4
3 Wrist-biting	4	19	1	6·6	2	12	0	0
4 Face-slapping and punching	5	24	1	6·6	1	6	0	0

activities were carried out, in a milder form, when the child appeared calm and happy. They then seemed to be more a time-filling or exploratory action, or possibly designed to attract notice from an adult. Head-banging and face-slapping also at times appeared to be compulsive habits that afforded some satisfaction to the child, but usually they were associated with disturbed periods. Whenever a child was engaged in persistent head-banging or face-slapping, it was found very difficult to break him from the activity, or to gain access at all, while the action was at its most intense. One boy (Christopher: Case History 5) brought up large bruises over his face by constant slapping. Another had banged his head so intensively that a ridge of calloused skin had developed on his forehead. Such extreme cases were limited to the psychotic group. Wrist-biting was often only transient and in some children appeared to be a reflex action, whenever they were frustrated. As a child improved he might go through the motions of biting without inflicting any damage at all.

OBSESSIONAL AND MANNERISTIC BEHAVIOUR (*Tables 8 and 9 below and p. 32*)

A large number of symptoms observed in the children at West Stowell reflected the obsessional nature of much of their behaviour, both in thought and action. It was this obsessiveness, together with various stereotyped mannerisms, which most clearly marked off the psychotic children from those suffering from subnormality and conduct disorders. It was interesting to note that in one or two children object-obsessions lessened as the child matured and improved,

TABLE 8 OBSESSIONAL BEHAVIOUR

	Psychotic		Psychotic and severely subnormal		Disturbed subnormal		Conduct disorder	
Total cases in category	21		15		17		18	
	N	%	N	%	N	%	N	%
1 Ritualistic patterns	9	43	5	33	0	0	1	5·7
2 Ritual questioning	6	29	2	13	1	6	0	0
3 Object-obsession	8	38	9	60	3	18	0	0
4 Subject-obsession	8	38	2	13	2	12	2	11·4

but were continued as subject-obsessions (i.e. interests associated with human beings) as the child developed communicative speech.

Ritualistic patterns of behaviour were individual to each child and were often of considerable complexity. One boy (Neville: Case History 11) went through the same pattern of activities whenever he returned from a home leave. He would look at the clock, dash off to the lavatory, urinate, have a drink of water, and then lie on the floor and kick his feet in the air, laughing loudly, after which he would quietly run off to watch from an upstairs window as his

D

father drove off in his car. Another (Roger: Case History 15) went through a long ritual of crawling about on the floor, out of sight and under tables, before accepting verbal, visual, or physical contact with the author. Ritual questioning, which was often associated with these behaviour patterns, was found almost entirely in the psychotic groups. The questioning tended to be on single or limited topics and was often associated with subject-obsessions. Time, place, and toilet matters were the most common topics:'Where do you live?' 'What time do you go home'? 'Who is on duty?' 'Is Mr X coming to tea?' 'When can I go to the toilet?' Such questions might be repeated many times, with increasing intensity and anxiety.

In some cases the questions were of a bizarre nature with no 'right' answer. One boy would ask questions such as 'Can I sleep out here tonight?' 'Can I hit you?' 'Will you hit me if I black your eye?' The answer 'No' led to renewed questioning, a 'Yes' led to a frightened 'No' or a puzzled 'Why?' but neither appeared to be in any way satisfying. Another child (Denis: Case History 7) asked obsessively about double white lines on the road; why they were there and who put them there, and would then extend this into other road matters, and finally would ask if people would be fined if the white lines were crossed.

Object-obsession was mainly in the form of a fascination with a particular mechanical object, especially clocks and torches, or a need for a security symbol. One boy (Richard: Case History 14) carried round two small wooden blocks which he clapped together, but would make do with any other two objects if they were not available. Another was content with a stick. Some would need a particular toy or piece of clothing. Later such children might turn to a topic as an obsession, especially as they developed speech. One psychotic boy (Andrew: Case History 1) became obsessed with aeroplanes and rockets, collecting pictures of them and drawing them himself. Later his interest turned to cathedrals, and later still he talked only of mountains and volcanoes.

All such behaviour was much more common in the psychotic children than in the other groups. It was especially among children with subject-obsessions that the so-called 'islets of ability' were seen. In some instances these were little more than flashes of interest shown by a very dull child. One psychotic boy aged 13 (Bobby: Case History 4), who had reasonable speech but little educational achievement, developed an interest in Roman Britain, learned a few facts, made some plasticine models, and soon developed an islet of ability in this sphere. In fact, his achievement was limited, but the interest shown was still remarkable and beyond his general level. It seemed to be associated with a good relationship with his teacher. A fundamental point appeared to be that this interest was self-chosen by him within the schoolroom. There were many other instances of a higher level of competence in self-selected tasks as against levels of achievements in formal settings and imposed activities.

There were cases where in a limited sphere a child showed above average ability. Andrew, the boy who showed an obsessive interest in cathedrals, could quickly draw an accurate representation of several of these and give details of height, age, and style. This same boy had an exceptional grasp of dates. He would ask visitors when their birthdays were and, if told the date of the month, would inform them of the day of the week on which their birthday fell in that year. A keenly developed time sense was noted in one or two other children. One boy, who was always asking about the time, would be able to tell it, accurately to within a few minutes, if asked, although he had no watch. The same boy had a great skill in map-reading, could place the counties of England on a blank map, and had a detailed knowledge of distances between local villages.

Most of the children with subject-obsessions did well. They were speaking children who had worked through the worst of their illness and were moving forward on a narrow front. One exception was a boy whose mental illness was so unremitting that his ritual questioning, and obsessions were a barrier between himself and an adult, yet even here a clarity of thought far above his general operating level would occasionally come through his obsessive talk, suggesting unrealizable potential.

MANNERISTIC ACTIVITIES (*Table 9, p. 32*)

Repetitive manneristic movements displayed singly or in patterns have already been discussed. Some children displayed several of these symptoms. Over half of both psychotic groups showed at least one, while they were notably absent in the conduct-disorder group. In this study a wide range of individual activities has been noted, provided that they were either common, frequent, or both. Most of the children showing massive stereotyped movements had been diagnosed as 'autistic'. Psychotic children showing none of these symptoms usually had behaviour patterns marked by the obsessional behaviour previously discussed. The four 'disturbed subnormals'

TABLE 9 MANNERISTIC ACTIVITIES

	Psychotic		Psychotic and severely subnormal		Disturbed subnormal		Conduct disorder
Total cases in category	21		15		17		18
	N	%	N	%	N	%	
Stereotyped repetitive movements of any sort	14	66	8	53	4	24	0
1 Finger-play	5	24	1	6·5	2	12	0
2 Flicking	3	15	2	13	1	6	0
3 Sifting and shaking	4	18	3	20	2	12	0
4 Strip-waving	2	9	2	13	0	0	0
5 Toy-rattling	3	15	2	13	1	6	0
6 Wall-picking	2	9	0	0	1	6	0
7 Paper-tearing	5	24	5	33	1	6	0
8 Posting	2	9	0	0	1	6	0
9 Sweeping	2	9	0	0	0	0	0

who showed this type of manneristic behaviour were exceptionally complicated cases, where the emotional disturbances had, at times, approached psychotic intensity.

As these manneristic activities seem of major importance in psychotic behaviour, nine are described in some detail below.

1. *Finger-play*

This covers a wide range of manneristic movement of the fingers, often carried out close to the eyes. One girl would flick her fingers up and down in front of her, without bothering to watch them for much of the time, as if the movement was pleasurable in itself. For other children the important element seemed to be to watch the finger movements, while some moved their hand from the wrist in action better described as hand-flapping. This movement has been included in this group where it was used in a similar way to other finger-play (e.g. where the child watched the flapping movement closely).

2. *Flicking*

The term 'flicking' is used to mean the act of sending particles of chalk, fluff, or dust into the air, and usually watching them float to the ground. It was not always clear whether the main aim of the activity was to watch the results, but this seemed likely, especially as most of the children who did this were also fond of watching bubbles float about. One boy (Guy: Case History 9) spent long periods absorbed in plucking wool from his pullover and flicking it up into the air. Another (Christopher: Case History 5) would slowly demolish a stick of chalk by flicking it away with his right thumb nail. Yet another would flick sand or dust, and his own spittle if there was nothing else to flick.

3. *Sifting and Shaking*

In many ways this activity was similar to the above. Sand was popular, and some children would spend hours tossing it up in front of their eyes or letting it run from one hand to another. One boy did the same with sugar at home, and would go beyond sifting it to scattering it about. An interesting variation was found in a psychotic and severely subnormal child (Roy: Case History 16), who spent much of his time in shaking small stones on a piece of paper. He would improvise shaking equipment from anything – a box and two or three balls, a handkerchief and wooden blocks, even breaking up larger toys where necessary.

4. *Strip-waving*

In one child this symptom seemed to combine an object-obsession with a manneristic activity. He was seldom to be seen without a long strip of paper, which he would wave much of the time, but carry even when he had finished waving. He liked to run along with the paper streaming out behind him in the wind, and would not put it down for other activities such as pony-riding. Another child (Christopher: Case History 5) used ribbon and would watch it from all angles as he skilfully waved it with deft wrist movements. In moments of disturbance, when he would slap his face constantly, a piece of ribbon was one of the few things that could distract him.

5. *Toy-rattling*

In some cases this seemed to reflect an unawareness of the point of the toy, but some children appeared to gain pleasure from the sound made by a toy when shaken, and one girl would tap a toy against her teeth with great satisfaction.

6. *Wall-picking*

Where this occurred it was often carried out with a persistence that amounted to destructiveness. One boy stripped his room at home of all its wallpaper, and at West Stowell would pick holes in the plaster of walls.

7. *Paper-tearing*

This was found in a number of psychotic children and varied considerably in intensity. Sometimes it appeared to be an aspect of destructive behaviour, but in other children the tearing was persistent and obsessional. One boy folded paper carefully and then tore it, and was always systematic in his approach. Some tore paper and apparently derived satisfaction from the act of tearing alone. Another tore paper in order to 'post' it, an action discussed below.

8. *Posting*

Though not frequently found, this symptom was a persistent one in the cases encountered in this study. One psychotic boy (Geoffrey: Case History 7) did little else for long periods of time, and was often so engrossed in his activity that he could not be distracted. He would post paper between floorboards, toys into holes in chairs, and twigs into hollow trees. If nothing else was available he would 'post' his own urine into cracks in the floor, and on a trip to the seaside he was very upset until he was able to 'post' sand into the spout of a tea-pot.

9. *Sweeping*

The most common form which this activity took was the brushing of dust along with the hand or a piece of paper. The importance of the symptom again lay largely in the persistent way the activity was carried out, with the child looking for dirt, dust, or sand so that he could sweep it, no matter where.

OBSESSIONAL PLAY (*Table 10*)

Most of the behaviour described in the previous section was 'abnormal' in type, but it has also been found that normal play is often pursued in an obsessional and perseverative manner. Most of the children studied enjoyed playing with water, but several pursued one activity involving water, with an obsessional interest, for long periods at a time. One boy siphoned water from a large bowl into a bucket. Another (Guy: Case History 9) would fill a plastic detergent-holder

TABLE 10 OBSESSIONAL PLAY

	Psychotic		Psychotic and severely subnormal		Disturbed subnormal		Conduct disorder
Total cases in	21		15		17		18
category	N	%	N	%	N	%	
1 Obsessional play	8	38	5	33	3	18	0
2 Jigsaws	4	19	0	0	0	0	0
3 Water-play	6	29	5	33	2	12	0
4 Mechanical objects	3	15	3	20	1	6	0

with water and squeeze it, watching the stream of water with delight. He would repeat this action over and over again for a morning or afternoon.

The more able children were encouraged to play with jigsaws, and for some the activity became perseverative. One boy (Roger: Case History 15) became familiar with all the jigsaws in the unit, and would maintain his interest by completing them upside down and matching the pieces by shape and feel, rather than by building up the picture. Mechanical objects were also great favourites with the children. Early histories of psychotic patients often referred to a fascination for electrical equipment, or a preference for a clock or torch over ordinary toys.

ADDITIONAL MISCELLANEOUS SYMPTOMS (*Table 11*)

Table 11 includes some further symptoms which were felt to be of interest but which were too varied to admit of classification without adding several more tables.

Grimacing and manneristic eye-movements were found in a number of children and often persisted after good progress had been made in several spheres. In some cases, the eye movements were

TABLE 11 ADDITIONAL MISCELLANEOUS SYMPTOMS

	Psychotic		Psychotic and severely subnormal		Disturbed subnormal		Conduct diso der	
Total cases in category	21		15		17		18	
	N	%	N	%	N	%	N	%
1 Grimacing	2	9	5	33	1	6	0	0
2 Manneristic eye-movement	4	18	4	26	4	24	0	0
3 Pica	4	18	2	13	2	12	1	5
4 Food fads	9	43	7	46	1	6	3	16
5 Regurgitation	3	14	2	13	2	12	0	0
6 Open masturbation	4	18	5	33	2	12	1	5
7 Exposure	3	14	2	13	0	0	2	11·4
8 Disturbed sleep	5	24	5	33	0	0	3	16
9 Nightmares	0	0	2	13	0	0	6	33
10 Using other person's hand as tool	3	14	2	13	2	12	0	0
11 Retentive memory	3	14	4	26	2	12	0	0

thought possibly to be indicative of brain damage or actual perceptual difficulties. Food fads were common in psychotic children, especially on admission, but tended to diminish very quickly. In some cases they were bizarre and involved a refusal to eat anything but a single chosen food. One boy ate only biscuits for some weeks. Another would eat vast amounts of corn flakes for breakfast but refused to eat anything else all day. Regurgitation was found mainly in severely subnormal children and was usually associated with smearing of faeces, incontinence, and general inaccessibility.

The use of an adult's hand as a tool to open doors or lift a toy was usually transitory, and associated with lack of speech when it persisted. This means of communication was used in preference to pointing or gesturing.

Much more investigation, both neurological and psychological, will be needed before it can be said with certainty that in psychotic children the retardation and the psychosis are both causally related to some form of brain dysfunction, although this seems an increasing possibility. The psychotic child, manifestly not subnormal in appearance, who displays a number of near-normal skills, could then be seen as operating on a subnormal level due to his mental illness. Certain of the symptoms described above were found both in children with a known organic illness and in those where no such condition had been discovered. If individual symptoms could be related to specific brain damage, a major step would have been taken towards understanding the causes of, and so ultimately finding treatment for, these conditions. It is hoped that something has been done in this study to clarify the symptom patterns and to relate them to different syndromes.

CHAPTER 4

Brain Damage in Psychotic and Severely Disturbed Children

The early histories of the 71 children in this study were carefully investigated and recorded. Many of the children seemed so disturbed that their conditions were thought to be partially organic, but a large number showed no physical abnormalities. Therefore, each case was studied looking for:

(i) evidence of brain damage or abnormal development, as manifested in abnormal EEG's, retarded bone-age, epilepsy, etc., and

(ii) factors that might have led to damage; e.g. difficult birth, brain infection, and severe trauma.

In the majority of cases, especially in the psychotic and severely subnormal group, there were factors suggestive of brain damage, even where the appearance of the child was normal. In the cases where there was no overt evidence of brain damage, the possibility of a physical underlay still seemed considerable in view of the intractability of the symptoms. Little support was found for theories of a purely reactive psychosis, although many of the conduct disorders seemed explicable in terms of a constitutional vulnerability and mishandling by parents or substitute parents. *Tables 12, 13,* and *14* (pp. 39, 40, 41) set out some of the more common causes of brain damage and the frequency of their occurrence in patients allocated to the four categories: psychotic, psychotic and severely subnormal, disturbed subnormal, and conduct disorders.

From *Table 12* below it can be seen that possible brain damage at birth was the most important single factor, and the relevant cases were therefore studied in detail, together with available information about birth position, mother's age, and other relevant factors.

Details of these findings are given below. The 'other serious illness' heading referred to in *Table 12* includes pyloric stenosis and unspecified pyrexial illness with convulsions, where the illness seemed possibly related to a deterioration in the child's condition. The congenital disorders were various. There was one female cretin, a case of cerebral palsy, a girl with Treacher Collins syndrome, and a boy diagnosed as suffering from 'congenital multiple neurological defects'. The category 'Other indications' is included to cover all cases

TABLE 12

Category	Birth trauma	Meningitis encephalitis	Gastro-enteritis or other serious illness	Congenital disorder	Serious fall	Other* indications	No evidence	Total
Psychotic	8	2	2	1	1	3	4	21
Psychotic and severely subnormal	10	0	3	0	0	1	1	15
Disturbed subnormal	4†	4	2	4	1	1	1‡	17
Conduct disorder	7	0	0	0	1	4	6§	18
Total	29	6	7	5	3	9	12	71

* I.e. where there is no apparent trauma but there is an abnormal EEG, bone-age, skull, etc.

† Includes one boy who is spastic.

‡ No information on early history, but there is a suggestion of very poor heredity.

§ Family history suggests a possible genetic factor in most of these cases.

where EEG, skull X-ray, or bone-age was suggestive of an organic condition but where there was no birth trauma, no later illness, and no injury.

Table 13 (p. 40) gives some indication of definite pointers to an organic condition. There is a considerable overlap of factors; e.g. an epileptic or a hemiplegic child will show an abnormal EEG if it is taken. The evidence here was limited so that the results are presented with no claim to a comprehensive investigation but as indicative of the range of defects from which these children may suffer. In considering bone-age, only those cases where retardation was more than two years have been included as relevant, but a full study showed that more than 50 per cent of the children X-rayed had a bone-age retarded by at least one year. Where there is 'no evidence' of organicity, this cannot be taken to indicate a reactive psychosis or conduct disorder. The 4 psychotic children with no evidence of organicity were so chaotic that there is much to suggest unknown brain damage. In the conduct disorders, the case histories suggest that a constitutional vulnerability, often hereditary, may be a factor, as well as a bad environment, when considering the importance of family background.

Before considering the nature of possible brain damage at birth,

TABLE 13

Category	Total in category	Abnormal EEG	Bone-age abnormal	Epileptic	Infantile convulsions	Hemiplegia, blindness, etc.	Large skull	Small skull	Total relative	
Psychotic	21	6	3*	2	0	2	4	1	18	86%
Psychotic and severely subnormal	15	3	6*	2	5	2	1	2	21	140%
Disturbed subnormal	17	2	1	5	1	5	0	4	18	106%
Conduct disorder	18	2	2	1	1*	2	1	0	9	50%

* One case was 2 years *above* average; all others were retarded.

the basic data about the births of all children for whom there was information were studied, and details of birth position, birth weight, and maternal age are given in the three following tables.

The basic information from these three tables was not expected to be very revealing, but one or two points emerge which are worthy of comment. First births made up two-thirds of the 'psychotic' category, as has been remarked by Kanner, Rimland, and others. Approximately one-third of all the children were under weight at birth and these were spread amongst all categories, but overweight children occurred mainly in the 'psychotic and severely subnormal' group and were associated with prolonged and difficult labour. The main interest in this part of the investigation lay in the frequency and severity of 'birth trauma', as it has often been suggested that brain

TABLE 14 BIRTH POSITION IN FAMILY

	First		Fourth +		Other		Not known		Total
	N	%	N	%	N	%	N	%	N
Psychotic	14	67	1	4	5	24	1	4	21
Psychotic and severely subnormal	7	49	0	—	8	53	0	—	15
Disturbed subnormal	5	29	3	18	8	47	1	6	17
Conduct disorder	7	39	2	11	7	39	2	11	18
Total	33		6		28		4		71

TABLE 15 BIRTH WEIGHT

	Under 5 lb.		5–6 lb.		7–8 lb.		9–10 lb.		Not known		Total
	N	%	N	%	N	%	N	%	N	%	N
Psychotic	1	4	5	24	11	52	1	4	3	12	21
Psychotic and severely subnormal	0	—	2	13	5	33	4	26	4	26	15
Disturbed subnormal	2	12	3	18	9	53	0	—	3	18	17
Conduct disorder	2	11	4	22	8	45	0	—	4	20	18
Total	5		14		33		5		14		71

TABLE 16 MOTHER'S AGE

	16–24		25–32		33–40		40+		Not known		Total
	N	%	N	%	N	%	N	%	N	%	N
Psychotic	8	38	4	47	5	23	1	4·5	3	13	21
Psychotic and severely subnormal	1	7	10	66	0	—	0	—	4	18	15
Disturbed subnormal	1	6	5	30	2	12	3	18	6	36	17
Conduct disorder	4	22	6	31	3	15	1	6	4	22	18
Total	14		25		10		5		17		71

damage at birth may be a factor in the development of psychosis and severe subnormality. Information was available for 61 patients, and these were studied. As 'birth trauma' seemed too loose a phrase to be of use, all the cases were divided into four categories:

1. *No known trauma.* This included prolonged but uncomplicated births that are accepted as 'normal', especially in first children; cases of mild jaundice that cleared spontaneously in a day or so; uncomplicated premature and post-mature births, where birth weight was not exceptionally low or high (i.e. below 6 lb. or above 9 lb.), and there were no apparent adverse effects on the child.

2. *Slight Stress.* This included premature births of up to a month, which were not apparently complicated in any other way; induced labour with normal delivery; and breech birth. Adverse effects were again possible, but not recorded or apparent at the time.

3. *Severe Stress.* Cases were included where damage seemed highly possible, but no specific adverse effects were mentioned in hospital reports available; also cases of persistent occipito-posterior and face presentation; and forceps delivery in difficult and prolonged labour.

4. *Manifest Trauma.* This included all cases where the patient had clearly been affected by a difficult birth; severe bruising; cyanosis; asphyxia; or any other obvious damage.

Basing the analysis on these categories, the following results appear (*Table 17*):

TABLE 17 BIRTH TRAUMA

	No trauma		Slight stress		Severe		Manifest		No details		Total
	N	%	N	%	N	%	N	%	N	%	N
Psychotic	10	48	2	9	3	14	3	14	3	14	21
Psychotic and severely subnormal	5	33	3	20	4	26	3	20	0	—	15
Disturbed subnormal	9	53	2	13	1	6	1	6	4	26	17
Conduct disorder	8	44	2	11	2	11	3	16	3	16	18
Total	32		9		10		10		10		71

These figures are suggestive of birth stress as a possible factor in the aetiology of psychosis and severe emotional disturbance. Nearly half of the patients for whom there was information had suffered a stressful birth, and, as shown in *Table 12* (p. 39), among those who had not, the condition was often explicable in terms of later damage, following a fall or brain infection. Five cases were congenital. Where there is a congenital condition or later brain damage, birth stress would not be especially expected, and was not in fact found. It was considered that a descriptive account of the birth stresses undergone by these children would add to the value of the figures above, and the cases are thus discussed in their four categories.

PSYCHOTIC

Information was available about 18 of the 21 children in this category, and 8 of these had had a stressful birth situation. Among the other 10 there were two prolonged but uncomplicated first births, one case of slight jaundice, one slightly premature birth, and two births that were three weeks postmature. All 10 were without complications.

Four of the 8 cases with a stressful birth situation were described as difficult and prolonged, requiring a forceps delivery and in one of these there was a report of asphyxiation which necessitated the use of an oxygen tent. There were 4 premature births; one was two months premature and weighed 5 lb.; a second was born at seven months after an induced labour; the third was jaundiced and placed in an oxygen tent. The fourth child was born by Caesarian section, and had to spend two weeks in an oxygen tent.

PSYCHOTIC AND SEVERELY SUBNORMAL

Details of the births of all 15 children in this category were accessible. Six births were described as 'prolonged and difficult', in 4 of which the baby was postmature and weighed above 9 lb. at birth. Five others entailed a forceps delivery, following which one girl was left badly bruised and jaundiced, and a boy had to be placed in an oxygen tent because of asphyxiation. Another boy was cyanosed at birth and later his fontanelles were slow to close. There was one face presentation and two of the births were premature, both babies weighing 5 lb.

43

DISTURBED SUBNORMAL

Of the 14 cases in this group where information was available, only 4 had had difficult births. One boy was three months premature and was spastic. Another was three months premature, a twin, and weighed only 3 lb. 4 oz. One girl was cyanosed, having been born with the cord around her neck, and another had a difficult labour followed by a forceps delivery. Among the other cases there were 4 congenital conditions, and 2 cases of respiratory failure in the first month following apparently normal births.

CONDUCT DISORDER

Information was available for 13 out of the 17 cases in this category, and there was indication of stress in 7 of these. One boy was severely jaundiced for three weeks, though birth had seemed normal. Another was severely asphyxiated and cyanosed and had to be placed in an oxygen tent. One girl was three months premature, weighed only 2 lb. 10 oz., and spent the first two months of her life in an incubator, after which she was discovered to be deaf though her intelligence was unimpaired. There was one breech birth and one premature birth following induced labour. Another birth was by forceps delivery following a surgical induction of labour because of the mother's toxaemia, and the last was a forceps delivery following a prolonged and difficult labour.

BONE-AGE

One possible indication of an organic condition, suggestive of a failure in maturational development rather than specific brain damage, is retarded bone-age. In this study the bone-age of 50 children was assessed by means of X-rays of the wrists. The results are shown below, not with any pretence to statistical significance but as a general pointer to a skeletal immaturity. Simon and Gillies ('Some Physical Characteristics of a Group of Psychotic Children') studied 44 psychotic patients at the Smith Hospital at Henley-on-Thames, England, and found a marked immaturity in their sample's skeletal age. The findings of this present study support theirs and suggest that bone immaturity may apply both to subnormal children and to those suffering from personality disorders.

The table below gives the findings of bone-age assessment on 50 West Stowell House children. They are divided into four categories:

1. *Normal*, i.e. within one year of chronological age
2. *Advanced* by one year or more
3. *Retarded* by one year or more
4. *Very retarded*, i.e. by two years or more.

Because of inevitable inaccuracy in measurement, only category 4 can be said to indicate any real abnormality, but the general trend towards retardation seems interesting.

TABLE 18 BONE-AGE

	Normal	Advanced	Retarded	Very retarded	Total
Psychotic	9	2	9	2	20
Psychotic and severely subnormal	3	2	8	4	13
Subnormal	1	2	6	1	9
Conduct disorder	2	0	6	2	8
Total	15	6	29	9	50

There was no relationship between retardation and a bad prognosis, and in fact the cases with advanced bone-age all did relatively poorly. None of the nine 'very retarded' had suffered a 'manifest birth trauma' or even 'severe stress', and only three had suffered slight stress, which suggested that in these cases specific brain damage was not as relevant as a failure in maturational development.

In this study no systematic testing of intelligence or educational achievements was carried out, and it was found that many of the tests carried out by others, prior to admission, were not in keeping with the child's condition later. In these circumstances no adequate appraisal of the relevance of measured intelligence or educational achievements has been attempted.

CHAPTER 5

The Early Development and Family Background of Psychotic and Severely Disturbed Children

In the study of childhood psychosis much interest has centred on the age at which the psychosis appears to develop. One important feature of the syndrome which Kanner named 'early infantile autism' was that withdrawal tendencies were noted in the first year of life, often starting with the child's failure to develop any anticipatory reflex to being picked up. Mahler differentiated a group of schizophrenic children whose psychotic behaviour began later, and was apparently related to excessive anxiety over separation from their mothers. Rimland has suggested that age of onset can be used as a criterion for distinguishing between 'infantile autism' and 'childhood schizophrenia'. We now look at age of onset, early milestones, and possible psychic trauma in the children treated at West Stowell House.

The majority of cases admitted and treated at West Stowell had outgrown their infant years before admission. They had already frequently been examined, admitted, and treated by other doctors and in hospitals. The parents had invariably been questioned, time and again, about their child's early development, and their management and circumstances at the time. The histories produced by them, after this process, tended to have hardened into certain forms which were often repetitions, judging from earlier available reports. Nevertheless, there were often discrepancies between these earlier reports and the parents' recollections which indicated, in many cases, disturbed and disturbing forms of baby and infant management. These had often been accepted by previous agencies without mentioning in what way intimate handling of the child had been affected. There might be a passing reference to repeated changes of house and setting due to peripatetic occupations by the father. In other cases nannies, each with very different qualities from each other and from the child's mother, had alternated with mother. Mother had not infrequently shared care with maternal or paternal grandparents, or even used daily-minding by a neighbour during the earlier months or years of the child's life. Mothers themselves might be diagnosed as neurotically or psychiatrically ill, in the available records, but there would be an absence of contemporary assessment of the mother's attitude to the child.

The confusional aspects of the experiences outlined above for the child scarcely need emphasizing, but records tersely mentioned the facts and said little, if anything, concerning the emotional state of the child. Arrested emotional development, with poor differentiation between inner and outer life, the rejection of objects, parental and inanimate, and the overvaluing of inner sensations were often unmentioned, although destructiveness might be noted. The personalities of the parents, even where they were hypersensitive, vulnerable, and anxiety-prone, were taken for granted, and not considered in the context of the problem. The first year or so of the child's life, as a consequence, might seem a peaceful and passive period, the symptoms of gross disturbance breaking through only later in the second or third year.

It was largely due to lack of detailed history over these early years that it was difficult to obtain accurate information for the purposes of current history-taking at the time of referral. Much of the basis for assessing the early psychodynamic elements had to be synthesized against the background of the parents' unreliable recollections, often coloured by rationalizations, on the one hand, and over-concise statements in paediatric reports, on the other. In the light of these difficulties, it has been thought best not to put too much confidence in either the recollections of parents, or the completeness of clinical notes taken at previous examinations. Assessment of current parental personalities, combined with study of domestic background on a retrospective basis, and the use of dynamic interpretative methods, strongly support major environmental stress as a causative element in the withdrawn illnesses of many of the patients who came for care and treatment to West Stowell House.

Taking age of onset first, the inherent difficulties in obtaining exact information immediately became obvious. It was finally decided to base figures on the age at which parents first recognized the problem. It is probable that a large number of the children were retarded from their early months, but usually the fact was not recognized until the child failed to walk or to develop speech. The earliest recognition of the problem therefore was at the point where behaviour was abnormal rather than retarded. *Table 19* shows the age at which parents recognized that a problem existed.

Earliest recognition of the problem in the psychotic cases was related to marked passivity, avoidance of contact with parents, or persistent rocking and head-banging. Early onset, however, was not limited to children who were presented for treatment as 'autistic',

TABLE 19 AGE WHEN PROBLEM WAS RECOGNIZED

	Psychotic		Psychotic and severely subnormal		Disturbed subnormal		Conduct disorder		Total
	N	%	N	%	N	%	N	%	N
Under 6 months	4	19	1	6·6	0	0	0	0	5
6–18 months	7	33	8	53	5	29·3	3	16·6	23
18–36 months	9	43	4	26	8	47·8	7	38·6	28
Over 3 years	1	5	2	13	4	23·5	8	44·4	15
Total	21		15		17		18		71

nor did the majority of 'autistic' patients show symptoms of withdrawal in their first year.

The numbers concerned throughout are small, and once again statistical validity cannot be claimed for percentages calculated, or comments made, on the tables. Nevertheless, it is noticeable in *Table 20*, for example, that 11 out of 36 cases later recognized as psychotic or psychotic and severely subnormal, i.e. approximately 30 per cent showed passivity and withdrawal during their first year of life, compared with only 2 out of 35 cases, i.e. under 6 per cent of disturbed subnormal children and children later showing conduct disorders. A lack of response to adults was similarly a predominating factor amongst the psychotic and psychotic and severely subnormal, with an added differentiation between the psychotic and the doubly handicapped that 43 per cent of the former exhibited this compared with 28 per cent of the latter. Overactivity was more than three times as common and head-banging more than twice as frequent among the psychotic, as compared with the severely subnormal psychotic infants.

The order of differences found here between the four categories of cases is more striking than that revealed in *Table 21* (p. 50) which covers walking, toilet control, and speech, except that speech difficulties are very much less common and severe among the patients suffering from conduct disorders.

ABNORMAL BEHAVIOUR IN FIRST YEAR OF LIFE (*Table 20*)

Table 20 refers to the number of cases in each of the four categories to which a particular form of abnormal behaviour applies. (N.B. The same case may occur more than once in the same column against different aspects of behaviour.)

It shows clearly some of the differences in development of the psychotic and the subnormal child.

TABLE 20 ABNORMAL BEHAVIOUR IN FIRST YEAR OF LIFE

	Psychotic		Psychotic and severely subnormal		Disturbed subnormal		Conduct disorder		Total
	N	%	N	%	N	%	N	%	N
Passivity and withdrawal	8	38	3	20	1	8	1	8	13
No response to adults	9	43	4	28·6	0	0	0	0	15
Overactivity or temper tantrums	4	19	1	6	0	0	0	0	5
Head-banging, rocking, or other manneristic behaviour	6	29	2	13	0	0	2	11	10
Total	21		15		17		18		

EARLY MILESTONES (*Table 21*)

The early milestones of each patient in the sample were also studied and classified as 'normal', 'late', or 'very late'. Retardation was found to be common to all groups, but motor retardation was more marked in the 'disturbed subnormal' and 'psychotic and severely subnormal' categories.

Note: 1. *Walking:*   Late   = after 18 months old
                               Very late = after 2 years
      2. *Toilet control:* Late   = after 2 years of age
                                Very late = after 3 years
      3. *Speech:*   Late   = after 2 years of age
                                Very late = after 3 years

TABLE 21 EARLY MILESTONES

		Psychotic		Psychotic and severely subnormal		Disturbed subnormal		Conduct disorder		Total
		N	%	N	%	N	%	N	%	N
No evidence available		1	5	0	—	1	6	6	—	8
Walking	Normal	12	57	6	40	4	24	6	33	23
	Late	8⎫	34	5⎫	60	7⎫	70	3⎫	33	23
	Very late	0⎭		4⎭		5⎭		3⎭		12
Toilet control	Normal	4	10	2	13	3	17	2	11	11
	Late	5⎫	71	3⎫	87	2⎫	77	4⎫	55	14
	Very late	11⎭		10⎭		11⎭		6⎭		38
Speech	Normal	4	19	1	6·6	2	12·5	5	27	12
	Late	4⎫	76	2⎫	93·4	5⎫	82·6	3⎫	38	14
	Very late	12⎭		12⎭		9⎭		4⎭		37
Total in group		21		15		17		18		71

Finally, the possibility of early psychic trauma was investigated under two main headings:

1. *Major trauma,* affecting the whole of the child's life, such as a broken home, prolonged institutionalization, or rejection by parents.
2. *Micro-trauma,* where there was an apparently excessive re-action to a minor emotional upset of the sort that occurs in the lives of most children.

MAJOR PSYCHIC TRAUMA

Thirteen of the 71 children in the study were illegitimate, and 3 of these were successfully adopted or fostered (in that the placement still survived, even though the conditions might not be ideal). Six other children either lost their parents or were deserted by them, so that they had to spend the bulk of their lives in institutions. In the table below, two main categories have been used: children who had

TABLE 22 MAJOR PSYCHIC TRAUMA

	Psychotic		Psychotic and severely subnormal		Disturbed subnormal		Conduct disorder	
Total in category	21		15		17		18	
	N	%	N	%	N	%	N	%
Illegitimate	3	14·3	0	0	2	12	0	44
Successfully adopted or fostered	2	9·5	0	0	0	0	1	5·5
Institutionalized most of life	1	4·75	1	6·6	6	35	7	38
Very poor home background	1	4·75	1	6·6	3	17·5	8	44
Good home, but rejected by parents	2	9·5	2	13·2	0	0	0	0

never had a home for most of their lives, and those who lived at home, but in very unsatisfactory conditions where they were maltreated, neglected, or had little contact with their parents. In this last group fall examples of 'good' homes, where the child was rejected by the parents, or one parent at least, and cared for by a nurse or relative. (N.B. The same case may occur more than once in the same column against different major traumata.)

MICRO-PSYCHIC TRAUMA

Three examples of possible micro-trauma were studied: hospitalization, the birth of a sibling, and a move of house. These had occurred in several cases in the sample. Cases were included only when the child's disturbed condition was said to have started or intensified following one of these occurrences. (N.B. The same case may occur more than once in the same column against different micro-psychic traumata.)

In contrast with the 'major trauma', these occurrences were found mainly in the case histories of the two psychotic groups. Hospitalization sometimes had very extreme results, in addition to common regressions in socialization and self-care. One boy screamed whenever he saw anyone in a white coat; another went rigid in bed at night after returning from hospital; and in two or three cases the child's reaction was either hostility to, or excessive dependence on, the mother. The birth of a sibling seemed usually to be a disturbing

TABLE 23 MICRO-PSYCHIC TRAUMA

	Psychotic	Psychotic and severely subnormal	Disturbed subnormal	Conduct disorder
Total in category	21	15	17	18
	N %	N %	N %	N %
Hospitalization	4 19	4 26	1 6	1 5·5
Birth of sibling	4 19	4 26	0 0	1 5·5
Move of house	4 19	2 13	0 0	0 0

factor because of its concomitant removal of the mother, whether physically in hospital, or emotionally in her concern over the new child. In some cases the reaction was aggression towards the new baby; in others a change in attitude towards the mother took place, as noted in the effects of hospitalization. In one child the family's move to a different house resulted in his refusal to enter the new home for some days; in others the reaction was not so direct but was still marked.

The role of parents in the cause and development of emotional disturbance in their children has been much discussed. Bowlby's work on the effect of maternal deprivation on mental health is now widely accepted. In the sphere of childhood psychosis, Kanner's early suggestion about the role of a 'refrigerator mother' has been taken up by other writers, such as Despert, but is not now so generally accepted.

The recently available work of Laing on family relationships of schizophrenic patients describes child/parent, parent/child, and child/sibling relationships of a shifting, confusing kind that could readily be seen to encourage emotional development problems in younger children as well as schizophrenia in older ones. The mystification of children which is implicit in uncertain handling, widely varying emotional attitudes to feeding, nursing, clothing, bathing, and toilet-training, and fluctuating rejection and acceptance of general conduct is a non-verbal parallel to the self-contradictory management that is Laing's 'praxis' (accepted practice) of the parents.

The nexus of Laing, the self-maintaining reciprocal setting in which the child finds himself during his first 12-24 months, could be seen to be a continuing pressure even if individual practices were modified or changed.

The mothers of many of the West Stowell psychotic patients seemed to hold individualistic and odd views about baby care and child-rearing. They would usually to some extent be supported in these, though mainly passively, by the fathers. Full revolt by the latter was uncommon, as were major disputes, but mothers' methods would be likely to change a little as a result of paternal doubts. For example, one mother believed that nursing and dandling the baby were wrong, and from the second month to about a year never made any physical contact while giving him a bottle or feeding him. Another allowed her child to rock and batter his head and cot for hours, believing that the child must be allowed to exhaust himself. In both cases, the fathers made feeble protests, feeling even more at a loss than the mothers. Nevertheless, they played a small part in personal intervention, showing unexpected physical interest, from time to time, when left in charge of the child. Weaning difficulties might be entirely given way to by one parent, and made an issue of by the other. Crying, restlessness, demands for affection, were often dealt with differently not only by each, but attitudes would be reversed in inconsequential and exaggerated ways according to mood. Where there were other children, brothers and sisters tended to act out parental attitudes, distorted by a mixture of childish acceptance of the deviant sibling, and limited understanding of the adults' requirements. As bizarre symptoms of withdrawal, obsessionalism, overactivity,

53

retardation, and lack of predictable responses developed in the patient, it is not surprising that the situation became intensified for all, not least for the patient.

Although, as can be seen from *Tables 24* and *25* (pp. 55, 56), a proportion of the parents of psychotic children suffered overt nervous or mental illness, the majority did not. They did, however, tend to be shy, emotionally oversensitive, and lacking in a sense of self-value. They had often had emotionally deprived or unhappy childhoods or adolescences and had frequently been the victims of dominating parents, achieved educational successes at school, and proceeded to professional or technical training. Social mobility, although usually upwards as 'young marrieds', caused further loss of self-confidence in the women, both as females and mothers. The need to explain their problem to themselves, control the incomprehensible, and avoid making mistakes, often led to stiff, unrealistic, impersonal attitudes of child management, aggravating problems that might have diminished had confident mothering been possible.

Individual personal factors could account, in some cases, for the failure of patients to adapt as well as their siblings. Sex, position amongst siblings, parental preferences, illness, chronological impact of events, are among elements capable of producing a permanently distorted setting leading to personality deviancy even in the absence of formal mental illness.

Some differences in the parents' personalities and endowments have been tabulated in conjunction with the diagnostic group of their child (see *Tables 24* and *25*). The relevance of subnormality or mental illness in a parent, for example, could be at least twofold. Firstly, the child is likely to inherit genetically biased difficulties. Secondly, such parents are unlikely to be able to handle their children adequately. This sort of background was found in several children with severe conduct disorders. Among the parents of psychotic children there was less direct evidence of mishandling or poor heredity, but many had a depressed and anxious air, which was borne out in an MMPI (Minnesota Multiphasic Personality Inventory) investigation. Some of this seemed likely to be the result of feelings of guilt and inadequacy over an exceptionally disturbed child, and often seemed to be an aggravating factor in the case, especially during the period before treatment. The possibility of a continuous pathological interaction between parent and child, such as Goldfarb posits, seems a real one, and treatment at West Stowell House has always concerned itself with the parents as well as the child.

In most cases, parental mishandling did not seem to be the sole cause of the psychosis, especially as possible organic factors lurked in the background. Mismanagement could be seen in some instances as playing a part in sharpening the condition that led to eventual hospitalization. Parental attitudes also seemed to have determined

TABLE 24 MENTAL STATE OF MOTHER

	Psychotic	Psychotic and severely subnormal	Disturbed subnormal	Conduct disorder
Hospitalized subnormal	1	0	1	3
Very dull and inadequate	1	1	3	5
Very disturbed, paranoid, or schizophrenic	0	1	0	3
Unstable/psychopathic	1	1	1	1
Treated neurotic	1*	1	1	0
Untreated neurotic	5	4	0	2
Not known	0	0	1	1
No outstanding abnormality	12* 57%	7 47%	10 60%	3* 17%
Total	21	15	17	18

* Includes one foster or adoptive parent

the nature of the psychosis to some degree, such as turning an over-active questing child into an aggressive destructive one. On the other hand, several parents had coped well from the beginning, and many came for help and guidance, trying to be supportive and accepting, once the immediate strain of coping with their child was shared. Parental attitudes and the mental states of parents were noted in all cases. Sometimes attitudes were very difficult to assess. In 32 cases, there was some degree of parental rejection. This occurred mainly in the conduct-disorder category, 13 out of 18 parents having rejected their child totally or partially.

The social setting in which patients were living at the time of referral was also studied. There were marked differences in the pattern of background. Using the national census classification, it was found that there was a preponderance of psychotic children in the first and second social classes, i.e. higher professional, and professional, and a preponderance of conduct disorders and disturbed and subnormal and severely subnormal children in the fourth and fifth, i.e. semi-skilled and unskilled manual workers. Although the

TABLE 25 MENTAL STATE OF FATHER

	Psychotic	Psychotic and severely subnormal	Disturbed subnormal	Conduct disorder
Hospitalized subnormal	0	0	0	0
Very dull and inadequate	0	0	0	2
Very disturbed, paranoid, or schizophrenic	1	0	0	0
Unstable/psychopathic	1	2	3	6
Treated neurotic	2*	0	0	0
Untreated neurotic	2*	1	0	0
Not known	2	0	4	3
No outstanding abnormality	13* 62%	12 80%	10* 60%	7 39%
Total	21	15	17	18

* Includes one foster or adoptive parent

sample is a small one, it is interesting to speculate on some elements which might fit in with the finding. Other workers have found that autistic children have turned up with more than expected frequency in the families of intellectual, academic, and technologically trained parents. A wide range of hypothetical constitutional possibilities associated with parental personalities suggests that this may be a factor in addition to day-to-day management. There is also the likelihood that the parents of such children will be aware of the deviation of their child's development, and not only seek help, but will also inquire about, or demand provisions for, treatment and care. It may also be that excessive feelings of failure to produce a normal child combined with social pressures from relatives and neighbours outweigh the material advantages available to the child in his own home. These elements appear in many of the case histories, and suggest strongly that such parents are unable to cope with their problems at home and, being aware of the resources available, use them.

The referral pattern in the case of conduct disorders and disturbed subnormals is different. In them, as well as rejection in some cases, there is often a considerable warmth in personal relationship, even if management of the child has been inconsistent and shown a considerable mixture of attitudes. Often referral of the case arose out of personal problems, such as broken family relationships, inadequate housing, poor neighbourhood resources, all or some of which led to a heightening of difficulties which became insupportable at home. The role played by social agencies in referral was often more direct than in the case of the psychotic groups.

There are manifestly many other factors which could be considered, including the possibility that psychotic children are less of a problem in the community generally than amongst self-aware professional groups, quite apart from the possibility of these having proportionately more psychotic children. The overall situation may also be affected by the possibility that the majority of the community is as yet unawakened to the problem of juvenile mental abnormality. It is interesting to speculate how mass media such as radio and television will affect this situation.

One difficulty in considering the mental state of parents is that many anxious and neurotic traits in parents have largely arisen from concern over their child. It was, therefore, decided to count as 'normal' all such people, and in addition any who had been described by terms such as 'inadequate' or 'dull' and yet who seemed to be coping reasonably well with life. Those who were counted as not normal included all hospitalized subnormals, all neurotics who had received treatment, and those who had been described as 'neurotic', 'subnormal', 'schizophrenic', or 'psychopathic', where their behaviour or physical condition supported the description. Thus a woman described as 'very neurotic', who had persistent asthma attacks and talked of being on the verge of a breakdown, would be included; a woman similarly described, who seemed to be able to run her home well and was only depressed over her child, would be excluded from this group, and counted as normal. Finally, six categories of adult mental disorder were selected, and these were studied in relation to the parents of the four categories of children.

In both psychotic groups the majority of parents showed no mental abnormalities, but there was a group of mothers who clearly found it difficult to cope. A tendency towards depression was noted among several of the parents tested on the MMPI. In such cases there seemed little doubt that the parents aggravated their child's condition to the extent that there were real doubts as to the possibility of a permanent home placement. In one extreme case a mother rejected her son as soon as she realized that he was not normal, and was herself later admitted to hospital after threatening to commit suicide. The child was manifestly brain-damaged, and there seems no reason to believe that the mother's attitude was a factor in his disturbance. On the other hand, another psychotic child adopted by a very anxious and inadequate couple, who were quite unable to manage him in his later behaviour, which was marked by constant questioning and strange obsessions, seems to have been at least partially affected by their poor support, and rejection.

Only 4 of the parents of the disturbed subnormal children in the sample could themselves be described as subnormal, but there were several others who were of only low average ability. Although in such cases a genetic element might be present, over half the children in this group were thought to have suffered organic brain damage resulting from birth trauma, or later encephalitis. Among the 18 children with conduct disorders, reactive elements seemed to be of importance, together with genetic factors. There were 14 mothers and fathers in this group who suffered from some form of mental disorder. Eight of the mothers were subnormal or very dull, and 6 of the fathers were said to show psychopathic tendencies. Poor heredity seemed to be a basic factor in many cases, and this was often aggravated by later emotional deprivation (5 of the children in this category had had no real contact with their parents) or by mismanagement. Three mothers had had prolonged periods of psychotic behaviour, entailing periods of hospital care in two cases. One of these claimed that her son was of divine birth, the father being a monster from the sea. Another talked convincingly of a conspiracy on the part of hospital and local authority officials against her and her son. The third was often in a state of paranoia, refusing to allow social workers to see her son. Such attitudes seemed likely to have an adverse effect on the children, and similar problems, in a lesser degree, were found in several other parents. In other cases, the whole family background was disturbed. One boy was the product of an incestuous relationship. Another was the illegitimate son of his mother by a man who subsequently impregnated both of his half-sisters.

Only 2 of the children with conduct disorders came from homes where both parents were stable and normal people. One of these children was thought to have suffered brain damage at birth, which was premature and resulted in asphyxia so that he spent several weeks in an oxygen tent. In the other case the pattern of development was near-psychotic in symptomatology, though following a more benign course, and was seen as a neurotic personality disorder, possibly of organic origin.

There was a history of mental illness in 18 of the families of the children studied and these were distributed evenly throughout the four categories. Two of the psychotic and severely disturbed children had siblings who were also disturbed, though less so than themselves. Four of the disturbed subnormal children and 4 children with conduct disorders had siblings with similar conditions.

CHAPTER 6

Child-centred Intensive Care

The general pattern and organization of West Stowell House have already been outlined above. We give now a more detailed description of the methods of care used.

Child-centred intensive care combines 'good parenting' with the special skills needed to care for mentally ill children, that is the provision of infant nurture, affection, tolerance, and structure according to the patient's human needs. Some of the children at West Stowell House showed arrested emotional development as in autism, juvenile schizophrenia, or hyperkinesis. In some, their emotional retardation was due to lack of appropriate early parenting and care, as in conduct disorders. Disturbed retarded children often show gross emotional retardation in addition to backwardness, and consequently have increased personal and social handicaps.

It is commonplace for all these children to be anxious, timid, suspicious, and obstinate, and to avoid new situations, whether these involve personal relationships, personal demands, or the acquisition of social skills such as self-feeding, dressing, toilet-training, or inhibiting compulsive self-centred activities. By the time they reached West Stowell House most patients had failed in acceptability to their parents, neighbourhood, school, or training centre, and gave the impression of viewing their environments as implicitly or explicitly dangerous. They seemed to expect little pleasure from dependency and had poor personal relationships as a result. Many demonstrated high demand for the personal attention of adults and were self-assertive to the point which seemed to suggest they found immediacy of action to be the overwhelming consideration. It was against such a background that child-centred intensive care was put into effect. This method of care attempts to diminish circumstances that promote anxiety, reinforces an atmosphere of happy acceptance of the children, and takes account of the fact that their attitudes arise partly from their special handicap and partly from their normal emotional human needs.

It also recognizes that children away from home have special problems, and that a hospital setting, even when attempting a non-hospital ethos, still carries its limitations. All children benefit from good parenting. Good parenting is affectionate, warm, and accepting. The social structuring it offers is within the capacity of the child to take, and does not return hostility, or bad behaviour, with rejection. It presents itself, in infant terms, through primary relationships, and in an accepting, affectionate, individualized way takes the child through his omnipotence, while the child introjects parental attitudes and develops the normal love-hate relationships. Holding, feeding, toileting, all play their normal role. At West Stowell House it was necessary to make this approach explicit, so powerful are the children's defences when they are first admitted. For adults to be smiling, never frowning, touching, holding, and making opportunities for contact was part of the setting. Affectionate talk is continuous in sitting-room, bedroom, or bathroom, even to children who are verbally non-communicating. Impulsive outbursts are treated as cries for help, and incontinence as a gesture needing attention. Anger and fearfulness are seen as aspects of the same problem, demonstrating that reassurance should be given. Movements and gestures by the adults are unhurried, and children are allowed to withdraw from time to time even if only to give them the repeated experience of being wanted. Giving children individual opportunities to make individual, long-standing relationships whenever possible with the same housemother and housefather enabled primary relationships to be re-established, and emotional growth to be restarted.

During the period of the study each family group in the unit consisted of between 8 and 10 children, and had its own housefather and housemother, usually a married couple. On days when the houseparents were not available, the group was looked after by staff well-known to the children, such as one of the play therapists or a houseparent from a neighbouring group. Houseparents had varied training and experience. Some were trained nurses, others experienced or qualified in residential child care. The basic requirements were a capacity to get on with children, provide 'personal emotional handles' for children to grasp, some previous experience in caring for children, and an open-minded willingness to learn. Older couples who have had children of their own have proved successful, and so have younger ones with some professional training.

Houseparents were mainly in-service trained and were briefed and guided throughout their work by the writer, who taught the basic principles and helped them to put these principles into practice in their own ways. Uniformity of approach and response to need were taught as being essential to reassure the children, as there were inevitably staff reliefs and changes. Regular seminars and case conferences were held to provide opportunities for the interchange of views and ideas between houseparents, psychiatrist, and nursing staff. It was found that communicating on this scale took up to about one-third of the consultant's available time and was necessary to co-ordinate family-group care, play therapy, and schooling. This was especially so during the first months of employment of new staff, or when new patients had been admitted.

A large part of each child's day was spent in his family group, although school or therapeutic play group would occupy four to five hours, five days a week when he mixed with children from other family groups. Older members of a group were encouraged to help the less able, and houseparents gave their groups individuality. Each group chose its own fruit and sweets every week, had an allowance for toys, and so studied the needs of its members. Clothes, soft furnishings, and detailed organization within the group, were within the choice of the houseparents so long as they conformed to the principles of treatment. At the same time, many measures were taken to preserve the child's individuality. Parental participation, with visits and home leaves, was strongly encouraged, and the possession of personal property, such as toys and clothes, was of great importance. Every child had its own clothes, whether provided by the unit or his parents, and special pains were taken to ensure that these were attractive and individual. All clothes were named to avoid the sharing so common in institutions, whether by accident or design. The more withdrawn and disturbed children often showed little awareness of this at first, but as they became more in touch, it was an important factor in their development of self-awareness and social ability. Every child received pocket money, and this was kept for him in a purse marked with his name. The more able children were taken to local shops by members of staff, and all the children used the unit's shop, where they were able to buy sweets and chocolate and so begin to be aware of personal choices.

Houseparents started the day with the children every morning at 7 a.m., getting them up and helping them to dress and wash. After this, children and houseparents would go together to their dining-room for breakfast. The meal came from the unit kitchen for serving, and houseparents served the children or let them serve themselves, according to ability. All meals are informal and houseparents sit at table with the children, helping them where necessary. The proper use of spoons, forks, and knives is encouraged, but not allowed to interfere with the meal being a pleasurable occasion. After the meal, older or more capable children help to clear the table, and even the younger ones learn to help by putting their plates on the service trolley. The children are then prepared for school or their play group. The physical contact which this entails has been found helpful in establishing a feeling of security in the children before they leave their houseparents. One of the houseparents will take the school children to their class, while the other takes the remaining children to the play groups. Those who have reached the stage of attending the local primary school leave earlier by hospital transport.

At lunchtime the children are welcomed back by their own adults and again have their meals together in their family dining-room. After this they play in their room, or one of the playrooms, until it is time for them to return to school. At the end of the afternoon the houseparents are waiting for them, and the children change out of school clothes and wash ready for tea. Tea is a relaxed meal lasting as long as the children feel inclined. When they are finished the meal is cleared away in a leisurely fashion, and the children are free to play with toys or go into the garden if the weather is good. During the next hour the houseparents encourage their children in whatever activities they choose. Some will draw, some do jigsaws, while others, more severely disturbed, may move about the room, or indulge in various manneristic activities if left to themselves. The houseparents give individual attention to these latter, encouraging them either to engage in more constructive activities or at least to accept being nursed so that a contact is made. Group activities are also encouraged, and often a general chase or rough and tumble will prove popular.

Between 6 p.m. and 7 p.m. the groups move upstairs for their baths. Each family group has its own bathroom and lavatory

63

arrangements so that the child's elementary needs can be catered for at the family-group level. Bathing is deliberately made a group affair and looked on as an occasion for enjoyment. On admission, children have been nervous of getting into a bath, but this fear usually soon disappears. The child's original fear and its overcoming in this way has often provided an opening for relationships. This has also applied to toilet-habit training. Houseparents encourage children into a routine that avoids anxiety, and a marked improvement in toilet habits is often observed. Bed-wetting and soiling are treated as natural occurrences, the consequences of which are easily put right. The diminution of anxiety resulting from this attitude often leads to the child largely rectifying the matter himself. It has been found that many such children are helped by the presence of adults, and some have been known to defecate only when their hands were held by a trusted adult.

After bathing, the children move on to their family's bedrooms. The older girls, who sleep separately, stay with their group until it is actually time for bed. The children then relax, spending a quiet time in their pyjamas and dressing-gowns talking to the staff or looking through picture books. A peaceful atmosphere is aimed at as a prelude to settling down for the night. There is a supper tray of milk and biscuits and by 8 p.m. the children are tucked up in bed and kissed goodnight by their houseparents, who then leave.

For about two years or so, soft background music was played at night. This led to quicker settling down and less bed-wetting. As staff became more confident, and their management more supportive, the music seemed to lose its value for the children, who settled well without it, and bed-wetting remained at a low level. A night nurse patrolled, raising some to avoid bed-wetting, and comforting any who could not sleep. A number of the children prior to admission had been reported as being very difficult at bedtime, but this behaviour tended to disappear quickly at West Stowell. On admission patients are naturally over-reactive, and often intimidated by residential care. Houseparents have found that time spent comforting them at bedtime has especially rewarding results. Children, overactive and unresponsive to settling procedures, may have to be moved temporarily to separate bedrooms or given mild sedation. Similar procedures are applied also to children going through disturbed periods, who may wake in the middle of the night, tear sheets, throw bedding out of the window, or wander along the corridors. Such children are usually in need of extra human contact, and the night nurse may have to nurse a child in her arms, take another on part of her rounds, or sit by a bed to give reassurance.

At weekends, the domestic pattern changes as there is no school and the therapeutic play groups stop. Instead, the children spend all their time in the family groups, with houseparents working extra hours to cover the mornings and afternoons. Usually one will work from 9 a.m. to 12 a.m. and the other from 1 p.m. to 4 p.m., while both are on duty from 7 a.m. to 9 a.m., 12 a.m. to 1 p.m. and 4 p.m. to 8 p.m. The aim is to make the weekend a relaxed family affair as it would be for normal children living at home. Sometimes houseparents off-duty would ease the burden on the others by taking one or two children back to their flat where they could look at books or listen to music while the houseparents relaxed as well. Such individual gestures are much enjoyed by the children. In summer all the children spend most of the day in the garden or go for walks with staff. In bad weather they stay in their family-group playroom, or go in for easily achieved projects with their houseparents. Each group has its own individual structure, atmosphere, and routine, but all try to provide the child with personal care such as he would get in a good home. The houseparents try to make every child feel that they are two people who belong to him in a special way, and are always there when needed. It is within this framework of security that stimulating social experiences and learning situations are introduced. Anxiety is further diminished by special efforts to ensure a tranquil atmosphere in the groups. Houseparents are helped by the in-service training not to respond to provocation with sharp answers or rejection, to avoid raising their voices, and always to show interest. They accept being tested out by the children as part of treatment.

With children as disturbed as those at West Stowell House, individual crises are liable to occur, and these sometimes trigger off group reactions. As a result a number of children may start screaming, some attacking others, some hiding or biting and slapping themselves. To deal with this, all individual disturbances are treated calmly. One houseparent will comfort the child concerned while the other helps the rest to carry on as if nothing important had happened. A broken cup, soiled pants, a temper tantrum, or an attack on another child are all accepted as something easily remedied.

When the child concerned has recovered his composure, he is encouraged to help the situation by picking up the cup he has broken or kissing the child he has hit. This has often been found useful in reassuring the transgressor, who may be puzzled and frightened by what he has done.

West Stowell House is organized so that punishment is not used. Misbehaviour is seen as a demonstration of a child's needs, and his management is concerned primarily with meeting these needs. If a child has a tantrum, as the result of tiredness and circumstances, he may be put to bed, but this would be in order to give needed rest and extra care, not to punish him. Someone would stay with him for a time so that he understood this. If one child attacks another, separation is necessary, but does not entail rejection of the attacker. Houseparents are encouraged to deal with aggression by giving immediate attention to the aggressor as well as comforting the victim, and so diminishing the anxiety, or feelings of rejection, that may have triggered off the attack. If attention is paid only to the child attacked, further personality difficulties in the aggressor are encouraged. However, with foresight, many such situations can be avoided and the atmosphere kept calm and reassuring. Aggression towards staff has often been a way of testing out their affection, and is seen to diminish when it is not met with counter-aggression. There are, naturally, occasions when a child is too disturbed to stay in his group and at such times the senior nursing staff takes the child out of his group and gives him special attention for a period. This may entail his sleeping away from, rather than in, the setting that disturbed him, and during the day he may spend much time being nursed, up and about, or in bed, rather than going into the more demanding atmosphere of a play group or school class.

Once a child's placing in a group is made it is rarely changed except for reasons concerned with either the child himself, or his peers. Each family group would contain a variety of abilities, conditions, and ages, and this has been found to provide stimulation, especially for the more withdrawn child. To give a clearer picture of the pattern of a family group, one of the groups in which a number of older children had been placed is described in detail as it was at the time of the study.

The group consisted of nine children, ranging in age from 5 to 13 years. Bobby (Case History 4), who was 13, and Andrew (Case

History 1), who was 10, had both been in the unit for over six years, and were now both improved to the extent of playing a part in helping the group as 'older brothers'. Andrew came to the unit as a 4-year-old autistic child, totally out of contact with adults, over-active, a violent head-banger, doubly incontinent, and without speech. He now attended the local school and was a lively talkative boy, with an obsessive interest in cathedrals and mountains. Bobby, too, had come a long way from the aggressive, tantrum-throwing child who was always running away, the chief reason for his admission. Both now appeared 'normal' for much of the time, but a small difficulty could still lead to regression at an infantile level. They had gained much from the presence of Pamela (Case History 12) and Joseph (Case History 10) who were both children of average intelligence with severe conduct disorders but basically normal patterns of personality. Pamela was 8 years old and severely deaf. She was in some ways now the most stable member of the group, and was aware of the odd nature of the behaviour of others, indignantly bringing this to the notice of the houseparents with exclamatory grunts and shrieks. Her houseparents had gained her confidence by continuously taking care to communicate to her with mouthed words and gestures, and to observe her responses carefully so as to minimize the frustrations inevitably arising from her handicap. Joseph (Case History 10) was a 9-year-old coloured boy who was admitted to West Stowell House for a year as a short-term admission. He tended very much to dominate the group and tried to use Bobby and Andrew as his henchmen. At first his aim was to stir up rebellion against the houseparents, but they gained his confidence and showed him how to find satisfaction in the role of protector of the younger members of the group against aggression from other groups. When Joseph came in he was very conscious of his different colour. At the children's home where he had been living and the school he had attended he had been aggressive and disruptive. It was his houseparents' understanding of his colour consciousness that helped them to make some real contact with him, and give him some of his first experience of being liked, and of being found useful.

Three of the other children showed the classical symptoms of 'autism'. They were attractive-looking children of intelligent appearance, blue eyes, and fair hair. None had developed speech, and all would be content to spend long periods in self-chosen activities such

67

as strip-waving, wool-plucking, and rocking. Arnold (Case History 2), the youngest, rocked for much of the time, sitting cross-legged if left alone. At first he met all adult approaches with puzzled and apprehensive looks, but gradually he had come to accept physical contact and would ask to be lifted up. His houseparents were hopeful that he might develop as well as Andrew, but so far he still seemed to have insufficient need to communicate to make speaking a worthwhile effort. Guy (Case History 9) and Christopher (Case History 5) were both older children, and remained fairly inaccessible after three or four years of intensive care. Neither had more than two or three words, and in both their psychotic mannerisms and indifference to adults had shown little apparent change over the years. Christopher had recently shown extra problems because of loss of interest in food, and persistent self-face-slapping which had resulted in extensive bruising. Guy, too, had periods of disturbance in which he picked at his face and shrieked and screamed at slight changes in his environment. He rejected most initial approaches from adults, and his houseparents had to accept many weeks of making quiet approaches to him before he was able to accept them.

Billy (Case History 3), another member of the group, was also 'autistic' in that he had little contact with adults, and tended to withdraw from emotional relationships, but his behaviour was marked mainly by overactivity, and a very low threshold of tolerance. The slightest frustration would send him into wild bouts of wrist-biting and face-slapping accompanied by short screams. On admission, he displayed a wide range of food fads, but with gentle encouragement he ate most of the food presented at meals, though he was still liable suddenly to hurl everything within reach across the room.

The ninth child, Glyn (Case History 8), was probably the most disturbed child in the group. He was 10 years old, verbal, and showed behaviour similar in many ways to that of an adult schizophrenic. He had phases in which he would tear his clothes, behave as though deluded, soil and smear persistently, and behave aggressively towards even familiar staff. This inevitably had a disturbing effect on the other children, and both Bobby and Andrew had been known to imitate him. He had little contact with the other children, and was rarely aggressive towards them. Even in quieter periods his persistent questioning was exhausting, and his houseparents had taken a long time reaching a way to deal with his needs without neglecting the other children.

It can be seen that the houseparents of such a group were concerned with nine children each of whom had major problems. In addition, the children's effect on each other raised further difficulties. If Guy became disturbed and screamed, Andrew was likely to be frightened and to act in a regressed way. If Glyn tore his clothes, Bobby might run away from the group to draw attention to himself. On the other hand, the children as a group often helped each other, took pleasure in family discipline and routine, and so made possible the houseparents' task. Pamela, Joseph, Bobby, and Andrew would help to feed and tidy up the more disturbed children, acting as 'big sister and brother'. In the absence of the permanent houseparents, the other children helped to maintain the group atmosphere and routine, with support from the other staff. The group just described was the one containing the more socialized children. Another group might have fewer psychotic and more subnormal children, and in such a group problems would be those relating more to primitive care such as feeding and toilet difficulties.

Child-centred intensive care has been applied with success not only to psychotic and disturbed subnormal children but also to re-active conduct disorders. With the latter, this approach has often broken down the resentful aggressive attitudes displayed on admission, by offering the child an understanding and acceptance he had never met before. In some cases response was such that within a matter of weeks symptoms such as aggression, bed-wetting, and exposure, which brought the child to the unit, had disappeared.

In a family-group system one difficulty that inevitably has to be faced is the effect on the children of staff changes. In the five years that the system had been operating at West Stowell House, up to the time of writing, seven sets of houseparents had been concerned with two groups, but one group had had the same houseparents throughout. For two periods of about six months, the system was maintained through the co-operation of play therapists and nursing staff, who undertook caring for the groups until new houseparents arrived. For a short period one group was run by part-time evening helpers assisting the permanent nursing staff. These periods have been useful in helping to consider the effects of staff changes and understaffing.

In many ways it has been surprising how well most of the children coped with these changes as long as the group was maintained in familiar surroundings and followed the same basic daily routine. Where regression occurred in some children it seems to have been more often associated with a disruption of interpersonal attitudes and timetables rather than with tensions arising from loss of individuals. The older children or less disturbed children who had reached the stage of forming dependent personal relationships with individual adults have shown the most disturbance when individuals have changed. With the younger and most disturbed children, the therapeutically orientated routine, and warm satisfying of needs, has seemed to be more important than the specific person providing care. Nevertheless among these, too, there were cases of a child missing mothering from an individual nurse: one boy of 8 years old, who had been receiving regular bedtime mothering from his housemother, became obsessively attached to a toy rabbit when she left suddenly. Another very withdrawn child missed the housefather who had developed a special relationship with him and had spent long periods in helping him to develop skills. This child regressed in interests, social competence, and toilet control when the member of staff left.

Most examples of regression have been short-lived and related more to the absence of houseparents than to the departure of a particular pair. One boy was noted to become markedly more relaxed in two periods following the departure of houseparents, as if he were aware that less demands would be made on him, and this was associated with a small but distinct regression towards more infantile behaviour. Another, disturbed by the absence of familiar staff, used to run off from his group, refusing to help with serving meals, or help younger children, as he had been doing. Two succeeding pairs of houseparents commented on this reaction, and described other patterns of disturbed reactions giving way to more dependent, approval-seeking behaviour as he lost suspicion of them. As long as the family groups have been maintained, most of the children have been able to cope with changes in staff. Groups have always been preserved for their self-stabilizing effect, even if they have had to be cared for by one member of staff only, rather than amalgamating them for administrative or nursing convenience. New staff, including part-time staff, were given training in what attitudes to adopt towards the children before joining a group, and this had ensured relatively consistent care in spite of changes. The study appears to show that the effects of staff changes can be minimized by the maintenance of routine and basic principles of management, and by ensuring that the 'bricks and mortar' at least do not change for the children. Where a well-planned transition between two sets of houseparents has been possible, the effects of change have been slight, and it seems likely that the best houseparents have not necessarily been those who have been 'missed' most.

In addition to the routine management, emphasis is also laid on what are called 'heightened experiences'. Many severely disturbed children, particularly autistic and schizophrenic children, appear withdrawn and unresponsive, but experience has shown that special occasions and activities can 'reach' them in the way they reach normal children. There is evidence to suggest that over-inhibition associated with excessive timidity may be largely responsible for their lack of response, and with this in mind, a pattern of special events was part of treatment.

Once a week, as long as the weather permits, the local Pony Club brings ponies for the children to ride, an experience most of them enjoy very much. The atmosphere of bustling activity on the arrival of the animals makes an exciting impact. Each pony has three women helpers, leading and teaching the child to ride. This degree of human involvement has helped to open up interpersonal contacts in some highly resistant children. Twice a week a remedial gymnast visits the unit and obtains good responses from even very withdrawn children by means of loud music, marching, and simple exercises. Older girls are encouraged to join the local Brownies or Guides, while the children who attend the village school always go with their class on all outings. Colour films of the children engaged in their various activities are shown to them regularly, and these stimulate interest and help them to identify themselves, sometimes providing them with a body image for the first time.

At Christmas the children join in all the usual festivities before they go on leave. They help to decorate the unit, make cards for their parents, and act in a nativity play organized by all the staff. Parties are held at regular intervals throughout the year. These entail

71

major changes in the routine of the patients' life. A large number of outside but fairly familiar, adults and children are invited, decorations are put up, party food is prepared, and a local 'beat group' engaged. For a few children their first party is highly stimulating and can be a frightening experience, as it may also be for a normal child. However, for most it is an important and exciting occasion to be anticipated and remembered. Some children seem to come into rapport when caught up in the music and laughter as if for a time they saw some point in being alive. It is hard to tell what direct effects such occasions have, but they demonstrate how easy it is to underestimate the capacity of even autistic children for normal pleasures. On occasions the whole unit goes on trips, to a nearby zoo or to the seaside, and these too have proved to be well worthwhile activities.

Individual members of staff are allowed, and encouraged, to take a child home alone to tea, or for an outing, as such periods of personal contact have been found useful in many cases. They also help the child to develop social awareness and experience, shopping, riding on a bus, eating with strangers, or in a café, all of which they may have had little experience of as a result of very disturbed behaviour at home or prolonged hospitalization. Houseparents and nursing staff have often found that such periods have provided a good opportunity to make some further advance with a very withdrawn child.

Day-to-day care and treatment include procedures to reinforce contact and heighten personal pleasure in participation. The gratuitous giving of sweets to the children by adults, as a way to increase pleasure, is part of their care. Staff interest, attempts to achieve personal goodwill and loving contact, are all emphasized by oral gratification. It accompanies nursing, caring and trying out new experiences. Birthday parties are also made occasions for specially pleasant experiences with adults, while illness, tiredness, accidents, and anxiety are used as opportunities to make contact, alleviate misery, and heighten reactions of pleasure with adults. Very overt evidence of affection and acceptance are routinely used for the same purpose, and persisted in even when there is no recognizable response for periods of weeks or months.

CHAPTER 7

Regressed Nurtural Care and Education

Child-centred intensive care provides a therapeutic background and regressed nurtural care provides basic treatment for the emotionally impoverished, detached, psychotic, and severely disturbed children at West Stowell House.

Regressed nurtural care is mainly carried out in two therapeutic play groups where the therapist is not primarily concerned with instruction or encouragement to learn, but with providing personal emotional contact at whatever level it is demanded of her by the patient. The younger and more severely disturbed children spend two sessions a day in these groups while the older and more able patients are at school. An atmosphere of affection in which there is a wide range of permissible attitudes and behaviour is cultivated. The affection is made obvious, the therapists showing consistent goodwill, interest, and concern. Toys, large and small, formal and informal, soft and hard, are at hand and used by therapist and child. Plastic materials, clay, plasticine, dough, and so on, also are available. Paper, paints, chalks, blackboarding, bricks, form boards, constructional toys and toys that can be taken to pieces, all play their part. A potty close at hand helps some children to feel toilet-secure.

For some it is the first extended time children have spent away from the effects of damaging adult pressures, which have often been expressed through aggressive, controlling attitudes. For a child of 7 years, operating emotionally at an 18-month-old level, acceptance at this level can lead to a beginning of, or the rediscovering of, supportive contact with an adult. Some children on admission are withdrawn and passive, while others are overactive, boisterous, and often aggressive, but avoiding relationships as surely as the withdrawn. The two therapeutic play groups cater for these contrasting types, and although different activities and equipment are found in

73

each, both are based on the same principles. In summer the two groups move into the gardens where they use the outdoor play equipment, but they are not in close physical proximity, and are not encouraged to amalgamate.

For the play therapists, the main aim is to use all available resources to establish forms of emotional contact with the child, and later to use this relationship to encourage the development of social habits and simple skills. At first contact may be limited to nursing, changing wet nappies, wiping running noses, and washing dirty hands. Transient contacts are reinforced by physical approaches in the form of hand-holding, cuddling, and prolonged nursing. A good supply of sweets, given out at frequent intervals, and at times of crisis, is found useful as a beginning to bring a child into more realistic contact with the therapists.

Some children make no spontaneous approaches and would be content to spend long periods alone, indulging in manneristic activities. With such children, frequent approaches are made by the therapist with insistent gestures of comforting or sharing sweets, biscuits, or drinks. In one play group children may be engaged in a number of obsessive activities. One may be face down on the floor determinedly posting bits of torn paper through a crack in the floor, another sitting in a window-seat rocking backwards and forwards, but watching the rest of the room. Another stands on the mantelpiece banging two bricks together, while a fourth waves a strip of paper and occasionally bangs his head with the back of his hand. In the corner of the room is a sand table, and under this a small girl may be found hiding with her dress up over her head, and next to it another girl, dribbling constantly, pushes a large broom round the room in a purposeful way. In the other group the scene, by contrast, may be one of noise and activity. One solid little boy leaps about waving strips of ribbon and making barking noises, and another runs up and down shouting and occasionally spitting. At times two may be engaged in a rough and tumble, but usually they ignore each other, apart from a sudden hair-pulling attack, or hostile reaction to being interrupted in an activity.

It is against such a background of the children's isolation that the play therapists work, using their experience and skill to bring them into some sort of relationship, and to attract them to more constructive play. At first a child may break off his activities only for long enough to take a sweet, but for many pleasure in relationships is gradually established, and they may then become exceptionally demanding and clinging. The therapist recognizes this as a vital step towards an independent interest in constructive play and learning, and uses it as an opportunity for starting speech. Time needs to be shared between those children demanding attention and the more withdrawn who need 'wooing'. Sometimes children make a passing contact with each other, but this is slight compared with contact with the therapist.

As the children come into better contact they begin to spend time in using painting materials, sorting, stacking, and matching building bricks, and playing lotto; at first in close contact with the therapist, later for short periods on their own. In the gardens swings, climbing toys, and slides provide opportunities for contact, and a see-saw helps a child to realize how another child can be used in play. Water is very popular, and when the paddling pool and garden hose are used there are opportunities for bringing a number of children to play in close proximity, if not actually with each other. In the gardens the children are able to run and climb, and will often entice staff into chasing them, thus beginning a personal approach to adults. Less deeply disturbed children who are admitted to the unit are initially placed in these groups for support and reassurance at a basic level until they feel confident in their new setting. Some move on to a formal group within a matter of weeks; others stay in a therapeutic play group for many months. The more seriously withdrawn children, those suffering from profound autism or severe subnormality with emotional disturbance, may spend two or three years in these groups, and they benefit from stimulation from the less disturbed children, in addition to the long familiarizing period with the therapist.

In the play groups the therapists are also concerned with two important aspects of maturation: the development of toilet control and of speech. On admission many children wet and soil constantly, often smearing and trying to eat their own faeces. Routine visits to the toilet are started as soon as the children are ready, and this usually results in a diminution of wetting and soiling within a matter of weeks. Before this stage the children are encouraged to look for a pot, and later to go to the lavatory. Success receives praise and attention, and only a few severely subnormal patients have failed to respond to this approach. For many parents, advances of this nature, after years of frustrated effort, are of great significance. Avoidance of over-emphasizing toilet routine has been found to maintain these improved toilet habits in the children, even while away from the unit.

Speech is encouraged even in very withdrawn children by the constant use of speech by the therapists, concentrating on the repetition of simple words: mum – mum – mum; dad – dad – dad; sweetie; yes; no; and so on. Often the first response to this comes with a repetition when the therapist is not directly involved. Nursery rhymes and object-naming follow and may lead to slowly developing speech. Speech may stay at an echolalic level, and some children have built up a wide vocabulary without ever moving beyond basic repetitions. In other cases there is progress to the use of direct speech. Understanding of speech, for a long time, has always preceded even the simplest use of speech, and even echolalia may well be seen by the child as the beginning of a verbal relationship in which he is risking himself in a new dimension. Once started, progress in communicating verbally as well as emotionally and educationally can be expected.

The end of regressed nurtural care management is reached when the patient has passed from withdrawal, through infantile dependence, to the point of being able to achieve an 'on demand' level in a range of activities, both social and educational.

Temporary return to regressed nurtural care after going on to a school group is routine, and practice has shown it to give a valuable emotional breathing space when there has been a transient breakdown of social capacity. Occasions also arise when children need especially supportive care. In such cases they will be taken from their group and given individual nursing, and baby management if necessary. This may take only a few hours, but has been extended over periods as long as six months.

It can be seen, therefore, that regressed nurtural care goes hand in hand with child-centred intensive care. A regressed-nurtural-care group will remove much anxiety and aggression. Many parents have unwittingly aggravated their child's condition by making demands he cannot fulfil or even understand. At West Stowell House the recognition of the child's real needs has usually reduced tension so that progress in personality development becomes a possibility for the first time, and drugs become unnecessary.

After a period of regressed nurtural care a child may move to nursery-school group activity in a group of 4 to 5 children. Entry to this group depends on his having reached a point of contact with adults, and the world around him, that leads to a desire to gain skills and an interest in carrying out tasks at the request of an adult. Most of the children feel that it is an achievement to join this group. The school rooms are in a separate building and so there is a marked difference in routine from attendance at a therapeutic play group. Chronological age is considered irrelevant, and the class may cover an age range of from 5 to 14 years, the youngest child being in no way the least able. The class has a daily pattern designed to give the children a feeling of security. The houseparents take their children to school and help them to settle. The teacher welcomes each child, greeting him by name, and asks him to find his own name in a box. He places it on a board on the wall and then takes a seat at the large central table around which the class, including the teacher, sit. The class then helps the teacher to choose the right day from cards, and this too is placed on a board on the wall.

After this introduction the children are encouraged in various constructive activities, usually individually, but sometimes as a group. Picture lotto, jigsaws, shape-matching, picture-naming, and the full range of nursery pre-reading activities are used according to the ability of the child. Sessions end with group activities such as sand and water play, or keeping time to familiar music with cymbals, tambourines, and other instruments. At all times a child is allowed to sit alone or play with a toy, if he chooses to, until he spontaneously takes an interest in another activity, or allows himself to be shown a new way of using his toy. Most of the children soon became interested and are eager to be shown the use of equipment, persevering longer than when an activity is forced on them. It is of the greatest importance that the emotional needs of the child should be kept in the forefront while he is at school.

The equipment is largely that of an ordinary nursery-school class, as is the atmosphere. Around the room are drawings by the children and other items of interest to them, including, for example, pictures of hair styles for a young boy fascinated by hair, and a battery-lighted doll's house for the subnormal boy who loves torches and bulbs, and who through this has learned how to connect batteries and switches. On first coming to the class, children begin with the simplest educational activities, many of which are familiar from the play groups. As soon as a development in ability is noticed the teacher encourages a small step further. For example, having successfully matched identical pictures, the child may then be encouraged to try more complex matching. Special use is made of objects and shapes that the child can feel, in view of the known preference of many psychotic children for tactile sensation. One boy made a major step forward in learning letters when his teacher made an alphabet out of sandpaper. The prime aim of the teacher was that he should succeed, enjoy learning, and so be motivated to further educational progress. When a child reaches the stage of being able to benefit from more formal classroom management he will move on to the next class, which is run on the lines of provision for the educationally subnormal. Here he will be expected to sit at a table or desk and eventually to move beyond 'play ways' and pre-reading activities, to attempt simple sums, copy-writing and reading. A child who needs it will have the individual attention of the teacher, making physical contact, even sitting on her lap if required, while the others carry on with their work, or come up to share the teacher with their classmate.

Emphasis is still on motivating the child to work, and usually the child is ready to respond. The teacher sometimes finds that it may take as much as a term to make sufficient contact with a child for educational progress to be seen. Once the relationship has been established, however, rapid progress may take place. All achievements, even if small, are rewarded with sweets, expressions of affection, and encouragement to try harder tasks. Special importance is attached to the development of social skills. A small shop where the children buy and sell is very popular and develops money sense. The teacher often takes the children for country walks during which they tend to talk more freely, relaxing in the different setting. The teachers in both classes apply the same general principles as the houseparents in child-centred intensive care. If the situation becomes too much and the child is upset he may return to the nursery class or therapeutic play group, for variable periods. This is taken as a matter of course, giving rise to little comment from the other children.

Children who have reached a fair level of attainment and self-discipline attend the local village primary school as a further stage in socialization before leaving West Stowell. There, they are expected to accept the demands of a normal classroom situation, although they are not required to produce much work at first. Often this move brings out more of the child's latent talents, and also brings about a more mature attitude. All the children who have reached this stage have been proud of their achievements, and have been upset if they have to return to the unit because of their behaviour.

Some children do not progress beyond the stage of a therapeutic play group, while others may reach the limit of their abilities in the nursery class. For those who reach the stage of attending the village school, the prognosis is often hopeful. Such children have tended to come from the 'psychotic' or 'conduct-disorder' groups, but often on admission there was no indication that they would ever reach this stage. Some children have attended the village school for up to three years, while living at West Stowell House, and when discharged have gone on to their home and an ordinary school, or sometimes to a day or boarding school for the educationally subnormal.

CHAPTER 8

Individual Medical Care and Parental Participation

On admission to West Stowell House, most children were receiving heavy medication. In nearly every case this was stopped, without ill-effect, and a truer picture of the child's condition obtained as a result. The exceptions were cases of epilepsy, which continued after admission. Some cases needed drug therapy on a temporary basis later, but even in these the dosage was usually much reduced from former amounts without ill-effect. During a period of six years drugs have rarely been found necessary apart from some routine medication for epileptics, who became worse if drugs were withdrawn, and at the time of writing only 2 out of the 26 children in the unit were receiving drugs. One boy received a small daily dose of anti-convulsant to control his epilepsy; another, who had recently been going through a very disturbed phase involving clothes-tearing and constant soiling, received a tranquillizer during the day and a sedative at night. Both were seen as temporary measures. Other children were given sedatives for short periods when exceptionally disturbed.

A number of cases improved materially after drugs were stopped. One boy was admitted from a children's hospital where, despite heavy tranquillization and sedation, he had been attacking younger children and frequently running away. Drugs were completely withdrawn on admission, with only transient withdrawal symptoms, and within three months he had calmed considerably under environmental care, was less overactive, and ran away only on rare occasions. Another patient, a girl of 8 years, was receiving large doses of tranquillizers before admission to control her overactivity and aggression. This was continued for a short time, combined with trials of other drugs. However, after two months, it was apparent that as long as she was receiving medication a proper understanding of her condition would be impossible. Drugs were, therefore, withdrawn. Her emotional needs became clearer, and within a few months she was showing a good response to regressed nurtural care, with much less aggressive and overactive behaviour.

Experience at West Stowell House suggests that when the environment is therapeutically orientated, with a stable, friendly atmosphere as the normal pattern, and without implicit or explicit threat, aggressive, impulsive, overactive behaviour does not appear to any great extent. It has also been found that the basic symptomatology of cases becomes clearer when it is uncomplicated by added reactiveness.

INDIVIDUAL PSYCHOTHERAPY

The range of required psychotherapy at West Stowell House is wide inasmuch as admission covers the spectrum of severe mental disorders in children from organic psychosis, autism, and juvenile schizophrenia, to conduct disorder in relatively intact children.

An underlying assumption in giving treatment is that even acutely disturbed children enjoy developing some human skills, from baby level upwards. They learn, for example, to make the appropriate associations between objects and the affective aspects of object relationships and normally enjoy extending them into the environment; they enjoy, too, developing self-awareness, physical and emotional, and self-management.

The prime objectives of individual psychotherapy of psychotic children are relatively simple to state. They are for the therapist to be included in the child's feeling system as a good object. From this position the therapist attempts to help the child to learn control and to channel relatively undifferentiated excitation into appropriate directions and constructive activities. Much depends on the personality and orientations of the psychiatrist, but the child's attitude to the individual therapy situation is crucial. It is often characterized by rejection of the setting, negativistic patterns of thinking, and physical overactivity. Often the therapist's first endeavour is to obtain inclusion in the child's basic system of object acceptances, and to try to establish a need in the child for contact. The problems of neurotically ill children are usually less severe. A need to relate is usually present, and communication is easier through speech or comprehensible symbolic attitudes or activities. Procedures to establish relationships, whether direct or through activities, follow normal patterns, rapport being established around the presented problem, manifest or covert. Materials for aggression and construction, symbolic and real, are available and play their usual parts in the development of the child/therapist relationship. Meanwhile, child-centred intensive care maintains support and provides a personal, social framework at a secondary level during treatment. Occasionally periods of regressed nurtural care are used to reinforce progress during individual psychotherapy. Children suffering from conduct disorders, in many cases showing aggressive acting-out in response to conscious or unconscious object loss, receive psychoanalytically orientated treatment aimed at working through the loss. Guilt feelings are shared and dissipated, and replaced by ego strengthening new relationships. Individual treatment may be shared with houseparents while the child, for example at pre-oedipal level, works out his conflicts again, using his substitute parents to overcome his fixated position regarding his emotional development.

Individual psychotherapy of the psychotic child in the playroom demands special settings in which the perceived environment is non-threatening. Objects should be familiar ones, tables, chairs, simple domestic equipment, and toys large and small, always kept in the same positions. A Wendy house, rocking horse, tricycle, and large tables with many small toys are useful items. Among the toys a dulcimer, simple jigsaw puzzles, constructional and dismantlable toys, paper and crayons, are all helpful. A blackboard firmly fixed, a toy cooking stove, toy pots and pans, and tea set, as well as dolls, dolls' pram and bed, are further items which are both reassuring and useful. Most of the toys are capable of many uses. They can be enjoyed by the child on his own, shared with the therapist, used symbolically, used in acting-out, used in an aberrant way, used to keep the therapist at bay, to fill in time, or to relive experiences that are otherwise uncommunicable. Many children will walk straight past the material to look out of the window, maintaining their backs to the setting. The therapist starts by making himself identifiable, slowly being noticed, or in certain cases identifying himself with an activity, such as dulcimer-playing, chalking, or doing a jigsaw puzzle, but not making direct demands on the patient.

Nearly all psychotic patients, especially at initial or early sessions, evade gaze contact, and this may continue even after transient touch

82

contact, shared activities, or the acceptance of sweets or biscuits. Invitation to contact, a hug, nursing on the lap, giving of a toy, or helping the patient on to rocking horse or tricycle may be acceptable for a long time before gaze contact. They seem afraid of their own feelings of aggression, anxious in case the environment returns their feelings. Moving from non-gaze to gaze contact may take place long after other activities and may be the first step towards a real relationship. Using the therapist first as a cuddling-machine, and later as an individual who is permitted to give nurture, allows introjection of what the therapist stands for, and subsequent easing of tension.

Forty-five-minute sessions, three or four times a week, usually with shortening periods of negativism coinciding with more contact, more shared acting-out, more control by the therapist in an increasingly verbal atmosphere, has been the pattern of response to treatment when successful. Speech, mainly by the therapist, but widely understood by the patient, played an increasing part and was sometimes responded to by echolalia which subsequently turned to purposeful speech. Negative transference with anger, violence, or destructiveness was worked through. The management of this transference might vary widely depending on the depth of the psychosis and the stage of the treatment. Enveloping the child in a controlling but manifestly unhostile embrace might be appropriate, or allowing some destruction might be necessary. Terminating the episode by change of activity, substitute interests, or escorting the child to a less stimulating milieu might be alternatives. Whether the acting-out was excitation leading to rage, limit-testing arising out of long-standing experiences of frustration, or misinterpretation of the setting for other reasons, each played a part in choosing the way of dealing with negatively phased therapeutic situations. Consistent therapeutic unhurriedness, and the acceptance of mutually understood non-acceptable behaviour, such as overactivity, screaming, spitting, urinating, passing flatus, or defecation, commonly lead to a cessation of these types of angry rejections of relationships, and a symbiotic point may be reached. Symbiotic attitudes give opportunities for the stimulations that children find pleasurable, and measures to diminish excessive dependence and stimulate self-identification, both at primary and secondary levels, are relatively easy to provide in the therapy room and the unit generally.

The profoundly psychotic patient often showed little direct response to individual psychotherapy, although social aggression seemed to lessen, and emotional resilience increased a little. Difficulties in understanding the explicit, let alone the implicit, aspects of the direct psychotherapeutic relationships were usually insuperable. Nevertheless, it is felt that the efforts made were not wholly wasted and might show results later. Judged by their response to therapy, and their later progress, disturbed subnormal children found fruitful the opportunities to relive through peaceful, pleasant contact experiences that had previously been dimly meaningful and frequently painful. Children with even gross conduct disorders readily make rapport, and implicit and explicit interpretation of attitudes, feelings, and behaviour are possible; while the psychotherapeutic relationship develops rapidly.

In cases of autism, where no speech is available, physical contact and oral gratification through sweets have often played a part, but many sessions of mutual acceptance will have been lived through before rapport at even such an elementary level is achieved.

Paul (Case History 13), a profoundly autistic child, would not only refuse eye contact across the width of the consulting-room but when offered sweets would seem to take no notice. If they were placed round the room within reach, he would get up some minutes later and apparently mindlessly go round the room, turn his back to where the sweets were, pick them up, and casually put them in his mouth. Once they were there he would as likely as not dribble them out again.

Roger (Case History 15) not only found it difficult to make eye contact but he would slide behind furniture and go through a twenty-minute ritual of coming closer to the therapist, worming his way on the floor, hiding behind one piece of furniture after another. He would be calling out 'What's the time?' while doing this. Sometimes he would roll a ball or a disc across the room for it to be returned to him. He enjoyed being spoken to, would accept sweets when offered, but for many months did not make spontaneous remarks other than obsessional repetitions. Psychotherapy in this case consisted of forty-minute sessions two or three times a week for two to three years, and reached the point of talking without the need for prolonged rituals.

Neville, aged 8 (Case History 11), after many months of relatively passive time-filling, standing by the sand tray asking anxious questions about what time it was, when it would be teatime, and when he would be going home on leave, became so excited during the sessions in spite of, or perhaps on account of, having his questions answered that he would develop a state of wild overactivity scattering sand all over the room, a degree of excitement he showed nowhere else. For some twenty to thirty sessions, Bobby (Case History 4), a juvenile psychotic with severe depressive trends and good speech, drew soldiers, ghosts, and witches. Although these were discussed at various levels of imagination and symbolism, he was unable to express his underlying anxieties about death. Nevertheless, he gained considerable support from the sessions in which death was talked about, and turned his inquiries to other interests which he dealt with in a similar obsessional way.

At the opposite end of the scale, well-verbalized children with strong anxiety feelings would express themselves both in words and drawing, and receive conventional psychotherapeutic help, eclectically based, and similar to that provided at child-guidance level.

In the years that treatment for juvenile psychosis and severe disturbance has been provided on an intensive basis at West Stowell House, it has become clear that direct consulting-room psychotherapy is useful chiefly in the context of an overall psychotherapeutic environmental approach. Individual sessions provide the child with additional opportunities to act out his inner tensions while receiving supportive acceptance, and management, in the family group. Often behaviour in the family group and the consulting-room differs, and this may be useful. Among the psychotic children it is the more accessible and those with some understanding of speech, if not use of it, who derive most benefit from individual sessions. Many of these indulge in ritual questioning which can be given full rein in an individual session. Neurotic children, especially, respond to individual psychotherapeutic procedures against the background of child-centred intensive care.

Although one cannot readily measure response to individual psychotherapy, the clinical impression is that a great deal may be going on even in the most inaccessible patients during individual psychotherapeutic sessions. Patterns of response tend to be different from those shown in group situations, and improvement may set in for unidentifiable reasons.

Individual psychotherapeutic sessions have been found essential not only for therapeutic purposes but also for the opportunities to assess and re-assess the patient's illness in conjunction with his reactions to child-centred intensive care and/or regressed nurtural care. Direct detailed knowledge is essential to the doctor. He must be able to contribute proportionately if he is to guide, support, and control a group form of treatment such as is practised at West Stowell House.

Since 1959 parental participation has been an essential part of treatment at West Stowell House. For many years admission has been made conditional on parents formally agreeing to take their child for holidays three times a year, as well as visiting and communicating regularly. If the child has no parents, the person or organization acting as parent is asked to give such an undertaking, while every effort is made by them to find a suitable foster home, or other accommodation, to which the child may eventually be discharged.

Szurek and Bettelheim in America, and others, have stated with authority, on the basis of their wide experience, that parental participation is to be avoided. They have aimed rather at replacing the parent, who is often seen by them as a major cause of the child's condition. At West Stowell House, however, it has been felt important to maintain contact, since, apart from any other consideration, in many cases the child will eventually leave hospital. The difficulties of arranging a lifetime of continuity of personal relationships such as is provided by natural parenthood are rarely surmountable, and helping parents, first as passive, and later as active, participators in treatment has proved well worthwhile. Even where a child's disturbance seems to be largely reactive to parental practice it has seemed important to try to reorientate the parents' attitudes and help the child in his family setting. This view has developed out of the writer's experience over the years and is based on observable changes in attitudes of parents towards their child, and their ability to cope with his problems when they are shared with the doctor and the staff of the unit.

In many cases it was the parents' inability to manage the child that precipitated admission, and at first, visits can be stressful experiences. Often the child will show apparent total indifference to his parents, or a reunion may be associated with tantrums and habit regression.

However, such stress has often been found to provide an opportunity for houseparents to effect a better relationship with the child, and this has later been transferred to the real parents. Meanwhile the opportunity to discuss their child's problems with the doctor and the houseparents, who have had his care, often results in the parents feeling less anxious, losing some of their feelings of guilt and inadequacy, and so becoming better able to sustain the distressing experience of their child's indifference or hostility. Parents are helped to see their child as potentially rewarding, however disturbed and abnormal he may be at the time.

Often within a year parents find that home leaves become pleasurable experiences, and in some cases big moves forward have occurred while the child has been away from West Stowell. All the children who are capable of relationships, or become capable of them, value their parents and look forward to all types of contact, even if they react sharply when they meet. The parents, too, are more able to cope with their child when relieved of the continuous responsibility and care of their severely handicapped child. By participating in his gradual progress they prepare themselves for the time when he will come home, and it is interesting to note that in most cases parents request the return of their child when he has made good progress.

A small minority of parents find their children so disturbing that they are totally resistant to seeing them, but this is uncommon and usually attended by special circumstances. Most of the children studied who had families that had not broken up before or after admission were gradually brought back into contact, in varying but significant degrees, with their parental settings.

Special additional help is given to parents who have special problems such as inadequate housing, a large family, or a home in a rural area where no supportive agencies are readily available for their child on discharge. Support from a social worker, when available, is usually welcomed, especially in the first months after discharge when the mother may have doubts over handling her child. A major problem in many areas is the lack of adequate day facilities or education for partially mentally handicapped children. Often places have to be obtained a year or more in advance, and few parents know how to set about arranging this. It has, therefore, always been seen as an essential part of treatment that satisfactory arrangements should be made before a patient is discharged. Protracted negotiations with local authorities have sometimes been necessary before a suitable placement is obtained. It has been found that such practical help is much appreciated by parents, and usually results in them being willing to do much more to co-operate with staff in helping their child. The value of parental participation has been seen over the years, in the more relaxed and competent manner in which they deal with their children, and in the relatively large number of children who have been discharged home, with confidence that they will not relapse.

CHAPTER 9

The Patients' Response to Treatment, and Conclusions

It is always difficult to assess results of treatment. Responses, symptomatic and general, have to be weighed against maturational changes that might, or might not, occur without treatment. This is especially so in long-term care that embraces as many aspects of a child's life as at West Stowell House. To give as useful a picture as possible, three methods of presentation have been used. First, individual case histories. These contain not only the available pre-admission information, the condition of the child on admission, and his general response to care, but also contemporary reports of symptoms and socialization, with follow-up notes as far as the spring of 1966 in the cases of discharged children. They have been provided to give a dynamic background and enable readers to see the time sequence of events, and the interplay between constitutional, environmental, and therapeutic factors. Tables, and other similar selections of material for study, cannot provide such a vivid picture. Second, all cases reviewed have been tabulated under the four diagnostic categories, and then classified as 'much improved', 'some improvement', or 'no improvement'. Third, all cases have been assessed on an eight-point prognostic scale of diminishing social viability. It is self-evident that 'success' ratings, in relationship to treatment, must depend to a large extent on the severity and quality of the illness and the degree of reversibility or arrestibility of the condition.

The eight points on the prognostic scales of diminishing social viability are as follows:

1. Able to go home (i.e. own home, substitute home, children's home) and attend ordinary school
2. Able to go home and attend a special school

3. Able to go home and attend a training centre
4. Unable to return home, but able to cope with a non-psychiatric placement such as a hostel, and attend a training centre
5. Not yet ready to leave hospital care, but likely eventually to progress to one of the conditions categorized 1 – 4
6. Likely to need psychiatric supervision for the rest of life, but to be able to live outside hospital, with community care, if sufficient supervision and protection are available
7. Unlikely ever to leave hospital, but able to carry out self-care and some sort of occupation, with guidance and control
8. Unlikely ever to leave hospital, and likely to need care on a permanent basis

Patients coming into categories 1 – 5 may be considered as 'social successes', i.e. as being able to return to community life, with some

TABLE 28 EIGHT-POINT PROGNOSIS SCALE

Prognosis	1	2	3	4	5	Total 1–5	6	7	8	Total 6–8
Psychotic	2	4	3	1	5	15	4	2	0	6
Psychotic and severely subnormal	0	0	1	0	1	2	8	3	2	13
Disturbed subnormal	0	0	3	1	3	7	6	2	2	10
Conduct disorder	5	12	0	0	1	18	0	0	0	0
Total	7	16	7	2	10	42	18	7	4	29

hope of a largely self-sufficient existence, although with supervision in some cases. Those in categories 6 – 8 have not responded as well, but may have made comparative progress, in view of their more intractable conditions.

Patients who have been discharged have been placed in the category approximating to their position on follow-up in May 1966, but with children currently receiving treatment it was necessary to predict their future progress to some extent. Category 5 was formulated to cover cases in need of further treatment at West Stowell for some considerable time, but who seemed likely, if current rates of progress were maintained, to go on to stages 1-4. With this category there must be uncertainty, as there may be later regression, failure of expected maturation, or the development of organic lesions, as has been noted in some cases of psychosis. *Table 28* above shows the prognosis on this eight-point scale for the 71 cases in the study, divided into the four diagnostic categories.

As will be seen from the table, children suffering from conduct disorders appear to have done best by the above criteria, and this may be largely because they were operating within the normal range of intelligence, and basic social competence, and were thus more open to the effects of therapeutically planned care and treatment. However, in many instances the effect of treatment on psychotic

TABLE 29 RESPONSE TO TREATMENT ON A THREE-POINT SCALE

	Discharged	Still treated	Much improved	Some improve-ment	No improve-ment	Total
Psychotic	7	14	8	7	6	21
Psychotic and severely subnormal	11	4	2	5	8	15
Disturbed subnormal	15	2	4	9	4	17
Conduct disorder	14	4	12	6	0	18
Total	47	24	26	27	18	71

children was more striking, as their initial positions seemed so bad, and had such poor prognoses. With many subnormal children the potential was essentially limited, but if they were able to reach that potential an element of improvement was achieved. To help to put matters in perspective, the degree of improvement in each case has been assessed on a broad, subjective three-point scale, the results being given in *Table 29*, from which it will be seen that by these standards disturbed subnormal patients have done relatively well.

Least success has been achieved in the treatment of psychotic and severely subnormal children, where a severe mental illness was combined with gross subnormality, possibly of common organic origin. On both scales these children proved least amenable to treatment.

They frequently showed extreme indifference to adults, and passivity, symptoms which were found to be most commonly tied to a poor prognosis.

As a development of the research study, follow-up investigations and reports were made on all patients discharged from the unit between April 1960 and April 1966. These numbered 47 in all.

The 47 patients were divided into the same four diagnostic categories, and their progress at West Stowell House assessed as 'much improved', 'some improvement', 'no improvement'. The numbers in each diagnostic category were 7 psychotic, 11 psychotic and

TABLE 30 RESPONSE TO TREATMENT OF DISCHARGED PATIENTS ON
A THREE-POINT SCALE

	Psychotic		Psychotic and severely subnormal		Disturbed subnormal		Conduct disorder	
		%		%		%		%
Much improved	4	57·1	1	9	4	27	11	78
Some improvement	1	14·3	4	36	7	46	3	22
No improvement	2	28·6	6	54	4	27	0	0
Total	7		11		15		14	

severely subnormal, 15 disturbed subnormal, and 14 conduct-disorder cases.

The initial placements of these 47 children on discharge were that 12 returned home and went to an ordinary school, 9 returned home and attended a training centre, 8 went to day or boarding special schools and 18 went on to another hospital or psychiatric unit. The findings in terms of their initial placement are presented above in *Table 30*.

Of the 12 patients who were discharged home and to ordinary school, all but 2 were rated 'much improved' after treatment at West Stowell. Two of the children had been diagnosed as 'psychotic' and the remaining 10 as 'conduct disorder', most of whom were considered to have had neurotic personality disorders.

Five were living at home with their natural parents, and of the remaining 7, 2 were living at home with foster parents, 2 were living in children's homes, and 3 in small 'family-group' foster homes as they had no homes to return to. All went initially to ordinary schools, usually into the 'C' stream of a secondary modern school.

All were investigated on a 'follow-up' basis in May 1966. This revealed a number of changes in their position educationally, although only 2 had caused trouble at home. One girl who was living in a small family-group home was attending a junior training centre, having been excluded from school. She was said to be well above the standard of other children at the centre. She was probably capable of education at educationally subnormal level and seemed to be the victim of inadequate facilities and rather poor local social agencies.

One boy was placed in a Rudolph Steiner School for maladjusted children after his foster parents had found that they could not cope with him full-time, but he was doing well there, and was returning to his foster parents for holidays. Another had been admitted to a hostel for maladjusted children when his mother went into a mental hospital, but he later returned home and went back to school where he was doing well at a retarded level. Yet another was still living at home but had been transferred from his local village school, at the age of 11, to a school for the educationally subnormal which he attended as a weekly boarder. One boy was still in a children's home and ordinary school, but had been in repeated trouble with the police.

Of the other 7, 1 was now working in a chain store, doing odd jobs, while the remaining 6 were still attending ordinary schools and coping well, though most were still backward educationally.

Three of the children reviewed had never been to school before in their lives, while the other 9 had all been excluded from school prior to admission to West Stowell. All were persistently uncontrollable, some had frequent temper tantrums, some showed unreasonable aggression, negativism, and major unpredictable episodes of contrary behaviour.

Of the 9 patients discharged home to attend training centres, 3 were mildly psychotic, 4 were disturbed subnormal young people, and 2 had been diagnosed as psychotic and severely subnormal. All started by making fairly easy initial adjustments at home.

On follow-up in May 1966 it was found that 1 boy had proved too difficult at home, and had been transferred to an adolescent unit at a subnormality hospital. Two older patients were attending at adult training centres. One boy discharged home to attend a junior training centre as 'not improved', after a year had suddenly responded to a Christmas party and started to move forward from his previous negative attitudes. The other 5 were all coping at home with varying degrees of success, and attending training centres, some regularly, some intermittently. The future of these patients seemed very bound up with their families, and they were likely to succeed in the future only in so far as they received support from them. In some respects they benefited most where the family's expectations were low, because they were accepted and loved despite their limitations, even though often their potential was not realized for want of pressure or incentive.

Eight patients were discharged to day or boarding special schools. Six had been diagnosed as 'conduct disorders', 1 as 'disturbed subnormal', and 1 as 'psychotic'. Four had been described as 'much improved', 4 as 'some improvement'. Two went home and attended day schools for the educationally subnormal, 2 went to residential schools for the educationally subnormal, 2 went to residential schools for the maladjusted, 1 to a residential unit for deaf and blind children, and 1 to an agricultural training school for adolescents of retarded personality. All the children at residential schools spent their holidays either at home or in a children's home.

In May 1966 3 of them had left their schools to work in sheltered employment. Of the other 5, 4 were doing well at their placements and responding well to education and training. One brain-damaged boy, now recognized as ineducable and epileptic, was receiving intensive drug treatment and seemed likely to be transferred to a subnormality hospital when he reached the age of 16. The 'special school' he was discharged to, in fact, turned out to be a hostel for subnormal and other brain-damaged children, where care rather than education was the primary concern.

Eighteen children had been discharged to other hospitals, and these were all in one sense 'failures', as the aim of treatment was always to get the child to a stage where he could cope in the community. On discharge, 8 had been rated as 'not improved', 7 as showing 'some improvement', and 3 as 'much improved'. Two of the children went to an adolescent hospital unit, and 16 to subnormality wards.

In the case of the 3 'much improved', all were in hospital for essentially 'social' reasons. One had been moved to a hospital in Liverpool to be nearer his mother, a widow living in a single room. He had recently started to have major epileptic fits. However, it was thought he should eventually be able to cope with a hostel and training-centre placement. Another, a girl who had suffered brain damage following encephalitis, was in hospital and doing well, but could not go home as her mother was dead and her father, living in an all male household, felt unable to cope with her care. Again a hostel place, if available, would have proved more suitable. The third, a boy, was in an adolescent unit, although capable of going home, because he had clashed with his unaccepting parents and so was placed in hospital on a 'temporary' basis because they could not cope with him. All these 3 children were capable of a better placement had home circumstances been more adequate.

The remaining 15 had all be diagnosed as 'disturbed subnormals' or 'psychotic and severely subnormal'. On the prognosis scale, only 1 was thought to have the potential to make sufficient progress eventually to leave hospital for sheltered employment, and 1 girl did better than expected and had left hospital to go to a hostel and was attending a training centre. Excluding these 2, the other 13 seemed unlikely ever to leave hospital. They represent the hard-core failures who, despite intensive treatment, are never likely to be viable in the community. All are severely subnormal, and all are suspected of a severe degree of brain damage. Evidence of this varied, but some idea of their physical conditions is indicated below.

3 were grossly abnormal EEG

4 are known epileptics

1 is an unsuccessfully treated cretin

1 is partially blind, and has a 'Parkinsonian' gait, and

1 has a severe right hemiplegia, and epilepsy

The remaining children suffered the after-effects of birth trauma and infective illness.

The children's response to treatment was shown, at varying speeds, in improved child/adult relationships, more effective socialization, and developing interest in the outside world. Relatively little movement in autistic and juvenile schizophrenic patients may occur during the first year, which appears to coincide with a prolonged watchful, withdrawn, self-interested period. The majority of even the most severely disturbed children, however, make considerable moves

95

within the next year, and only a most inaccessible minority appear to resist this. If no move is made during this period there is relatively little expectation of success over the next two years. In general, where the mental illness of the patient is not an aspect of a progressive physical condition, time and maturation is on the side of the patient. Children with conduct disorders and disturbed subnormal children tended to show response much more readily than the other two groups.

Speech retardation or total absence of speech is a frequent finding, especially amongst autistic and chaotic children, and is a continuing brake on social development and education. Even if gained, it is usually very late and limited, and there is considerable variation in the speed and readiness of progress and use. It appears as if many children who have learned to do without speech find it no longer worth while to learn it, and it is advisable not to equate success in treatment too closely with speech attainments, since important personal and social development continues even in its absence. Perhaps because speech is a basic method of communication there appeared to be a direct relationship between the patient's lack of interest in relating during his early years and the lack of development of speech. As relationships improved with treatment, attempts at speech were made, but it continued to lag well behind personal and social developments in every case.

These findings would appear to indicate that relatively short periods of treatment with child-centred intensive care methods, combined with regressed nurtural care at suitable levels, would be beneficial in the care and treatment of other emotionally deprived children who have lacked or failed to use earlier opportunities to make satisfactory child/adult relationships, and have drawn attention to themselves later by personal or social inadequacy leading to institutional care in children's homes, Approved Schools, or hospital wards.

On the educational side, satisfactory teacher/child situations developed more quickly where children had been able to make helpful relationships in earlier stages of their treatment at West Stowell. Autistic children, juvenile schizophrenics, and severely disturbed young children generally, benefited from considerable periods of therapy in the regressed nurtural care group and were able to make teacher/group relationships which were also transferable to new teachers at later stages.

96

Education and skill development, in its own right, has a manifest and important part to play, especially with the less psychotic child. Although educational progress was usually secondary to relationship development, sometimes the two moved together, relationships developing out of pupil and teacher reaching rapport through the indirect teaching contact. This finding can be generalized to children in special schools for the maladjusted, retarded, and handicapped, and also to teacher/pupil relationships in ordinary schools where individual children have difficulties in establishing confident relationships. On the other hand, new skills, as ways of extending abilities and satisfactions, outside of a relationship, did not appear to be important to very withdrawn, psychotic, or neurotically ill children.

A study of symptomatology in relationship to the main categories used throughout this book suggests that there is a range of psychotic symptoms that differentiate psychotic children from even the most disturbed non-psychotic children, and they are often more specific than the generalities used in Creak's Nine Points. There often appeared also to be a close similarity in symptoms between psychotic children with alert expression, good physical agility, and general overactive qualities, i.e. the autistic, and the psychotic severely subnormal child. Disturbed subnormal children and children suffering from conduct disorders rarely showed long-sustained 'psychotic' symptoms even when grossly disturbed.

All the cases described in this book are severe examples, and purely reactive causes for their conditions seem improbable. Further study, both neurological and psychological, is required to assess this impression, which is the result of intensive treatment and observation. It is possible that less severely afflicted children present different therapeutic problems with conditions more amenable to less intensive measures of care.

Concerning the parents of the children, the relatively detailed sharing of information and responsibility between doctor, staff, and parents as part of the management of a child's illness at West Stowell House appears to have been, in many cases, the first time that they had been brought into a prolonged constructive relationship with skilled personnel. This frequently led to renewed efforts on their part, better understanding, and a desire to participate. Although it is not possible to draw any definite conclusions regarding the mental conditions, constitutional traits, or genetic endowments

97

of parents in relationship to the illnesses of their children, there appeared to be a great deal of emotional instability at neurotic and psychotic level in many cases, and it is possible to suggest that many of the patients suffered from vulnerable heredities often associated with inappropriate management.

Most of the patients came from the extremes of the social scale. This distribution may be the result of many factors. Children from national-census groups 1 and 2, chiefly psychotic and autistic cases, have been referred on account of their relatively high frequency in these groups, but probably also because their parents considered their children had major treatment needs. On the other hand, groups 4 and 5 usually found residential treatment was necessary due to lack of facilities and opportunities available at home, or in local authority provisions, and in social agencies, such as Mental Welfare Departments and schools. These are impressions, and a social-work research programme would be required to clarify the situation.

The staff at West Stowell House found the children's individual responses to their goodwill and expertise rewarding, enabling them to sustain disappointments, long hours, and arduous duties. Their acceptance of the principles of treatment, and the manifest response of the patients, and their parents, diminished the inherent tensions and frustrations of the day-to-day situations. These circumstances should be repeatable elsewhere, providing that adequate constructive support and leadership are available to residential staff and that adequate recognition of their responsibility and contribution to such demanding work is given.

PLANNING A UNIT

The work at West Stowell House was both helped and to some extent hindered by the building in which it was done. It is a large country house which had minimal building modifications made to it. This made extra demands on staff and children as it was not partitioned, and there were no major practical boundaries between the three family groups. On the other hand, the domestic proportions of the rooms made it easier to maintain a family atmosphere. Broad stairs and corridors gave a spacious feeling, and the variety of the room shapes and 'nooks and crannies' provided a richness of atmosphere that gave advantages, although it made supervision more difficult.

It was originally considered that it might be helpful to give a detailed plan for guidance in setting up a treatment unit, but this was abandoned. There are many ways in which a unit of 24–28 beds for severely disturbed children in groups of fours, sixes, or sevens, or even eights or nines can be organized, and it would be invidious to suggest any single plan as the best. On the other hand, certain elements need to be borne in mind when plans are made for the setting up of a unit for the treatment of psychotic and severely disturbed children in small or 'family' groups. The group settings should be well insulated, one from the other, from the point of view of both sound and interference. The proportions of the rooms should be generous and domestic rather than institutional. Bedrooms should be for not more than 4 children and preferably for ones and twos. There should be sufficient variety of sleeping accommodation in each group for it to be possible for older children, as they develop physically and personally, to be given privacy. Washing, bathing, and toilet accommodation should be at an intimate level and not, as is frequently the case, dealt with by rows of basins and stalls. Playroom and dining-room can well share the same space as this would be an extension of the way the majority of children live at home, and should be at a reasonable distance from sleeping accommodation. Most children are accustomed either to going upstairs to sleep, or to the other end of the house if it is a bungalow. Building finishes, switch and tap positions, furnishings, and general equipment should all be child-proof!

Play space, both with hard surface and grass areas, should be available to each family group, as well as a large common area in which combined games, wider freedom, and general activities can be carried out. An internal space for congregation for general activities, meeting on the way to school, or therapeutic group work is also very helpful. It was found to be an advantage to have two regressed nurtural care rooms in close contact with the family areas, in contrast with having the school building outside. Medical and nursing rooms should be within the same space as the family groups. This gives a 'natural' feel regarding medical and nursing care. Psychotic and severely disturbed children have a greater tendency even than other children to neglect self-care in the open air, getting muddier and wetter, and often damaging themselves by ignoring dangers. A covered outside play area, with hard surface, is therefore

99

required as well. This enables children to work off energies, using wheeled toys like tricycles, scooters, and bicycles, or running, playing with balls, remedial gymnastics, or other physical activities when the weather makes outdoor activities undesirable. The lack of such an area has been felt at West Stowell, and it is probable that a considerable amount of extra acting-out behaviour has resulted from suppressed physical energy. Not only should the covered play area be big enough for the activities described above, but it should also be large enough to take more than one group at a time. The school building proper should be at some physical separation from the unit so that children who graduate to school can appear to 'go' to school. This acts as a satisfaction for them, and an encouragement for other children.

A continuing overriding element in the proper care of severely disturbed and mentally ill children is seeing them as individuals, and refraining from putting them together in large groups for any intimate management purpose. It is in this sense, as well, that the physical separation implicit in bricks and mortar is especially important, so that amalgamation of groups as a matter of convenience, organizational or administrative, is made as near impracticable as possible.

It is common sense that staff concerned in the care of children cannot make supportive dependable relationships with them if they are not given real opportunities to do so. This is especially so with children such as those at West Stowell. They make relationships less readily and consequently need even more time in contact with staff than is usually the case. As a consequence, basic staff, group houseparents, need to be permanently appointed to their groups with the same regularly appearing relieving staff. A minimum staff ratio of 2 adults on full duty with 8 children at all material times is essential. There should preferably be other staff available within easy reach who can act as 'trouble-shooters' when necessary or give more individual care than is possible on the minimum staffing ratio. The inevitable staff changes due to resignations, student training, and similar unavoidable interferences with continuity need to be minimized and not added to by the usual rotations of duty as in most hospitals. This may require special administrative reorganization as an additional problem in the treatment of the psychotic and severely disturbed child. Without the establishment of good personal

100

relationships by the child, a great part of his potential for recovery will not be tapped, and the other measures taken for his benefit – special accommodation, therapeutic sessions, training, education, and medication – will largely fail and be wasted.

PART II

Case Histories

CONTENTS

*P = psychotic   †1 = much improved
CD = conduct disorder   2 = some improvement
SSN = severely subnormal   3 = no improvement

1. ANDREW

Born: 4 December 1956

Reason for admission: 'autistic' child, very overactive and withdrawn, with frequent temper tantrums and violent head-banging when frustrated

Height: 3 ft 1½ in   Weight: 2 st 2 lb 4 oz

IQ: not tested

Skull X-ray: normal, but large head circumference

Bone-age: *c.* 3 years when 5½

Treatment: regressed nurtural care

March–December 1959: individual nursing

January 1960–March 1961: small play group for young children

April 1961–February 1962: therapeutic play group; child-centred intensive care in family group

February 1962–July 1964: school classes at West Stowell

September 1964 onwards: local village school

Andrew was referred to West Stowell House in March 1959. Diagnosis was severe infantile psychosis; prognosis was very poor. At home he was destructive, and his adoptive parents were finding him hard to cope with, especially since their elder daughter was seriously disturbed by his behaviour. He was the illegitimate child of two young and healthy people, both serving in the Forces at the time. During pregnancy his mother had periods of abdominal pain and a slight antepartum haemorrhage. His birth was five weeks premature and followed a surgical induction of labour, but was said to have been normal and easy. Andrew was a healthy baby and weighed 5 lb 2 oz. He was weaned and discharged from hospital on the fourteenth day. Andrew's mother wished to marry another man, who would not accept him, and so 2-months-old Andrew was placed with a couple who had already successfully adopted a girl.

Initially he showed no interest in, or dependence on, his adoptive mother. Though she tried to get him to use a pot from the age of 3 months, he was still not toilet-trained when admitted to West Stowell. His milestones were normal, but by the time he was 1 year old he was spending much of his time kneeling face down in his pram or cot and rocking violently. He made no contact with other children apart from his adopted sister, who was three years older. At 2 years old Andrew was smacking his face and banging his head for much of the time, often bruising himself severely. He could utter only speech sounds, but would draw attention to what he wanted by leading people to the object in question. It gradually became clear that he was very retarded. A consultant paediatrician remarked that Andrew's appearance was not that of a typical retarded child, and although slightly below average in height, he had a healthy and intelligent appearance.

His mental state continued, and in September 1958 he was referred to a children's psychiatrist for investigation of possible psychosis. For some months Andrew had had a number of periods in which he appeared lethargic, lying still and blinking for some of the time. He appeared vague and inaccessible, although he often seemed very aware of what was going on around him. Bouts of rage and head-banging continued. He refused to walk on the floor but could walk and climb effectively over bed or settee. The psychiatrist considered him a typical and severe example of psychotic disorder. In view of the early onset and the severity of the case, the prognosis seemed bad, and Andrew was put on the waiting list for admission to a children's psychiatric unit. At home he made little progress, and he was still so destructive that his parents began to react to the strain of coping with him while his sister, now aged 5 years, was becoming seriously disturbed by his condition. Hence an application was made for a place at West Stowell House, and he was admitted in March 1959.

Andrew's adoptive father is a surveyor. He seemed very concerned about Andrew, though somewhat defensive and uncertain. His wife had been described as a rigid and insecure woman, but both parents proved very co-operative throughout treatment.

Andrew was a small intelligent-looking child, the skin on his forehead broken from continuous head-banging, and his face bruised and swollen where he had smacked himself. He could not speak and appeared unable to communicate by gesture. He had to be fed and dressed, and was doubly incontinent. He was very unco-operative and would scream at the slightest provocation. He displayed no sign of affection for any particular person but would cling desperately to anyone holding him. If he were put down suddenly, he screamed and began to bang his head. In the first six months after admission he began slowly to take some interest in his surroundings and to show

106

some attachment to those staff whom he saw regularly. Initially he had struggled desperately against being bathed but later accepted it as a pleasurable experience. He remained very dependent on direct physical contact but now used staff to fulfil his needs, guiding their hands to get what he wanted. His management of toys was intelligent and persistent, and he would remain absorbed in an activity for some time, making small explosive noises to himself all the time. He reacted very sharply, with a loud cry, to any attempts to interfere with his play. By December 1959 he was ready to be placed in a small play group with other young children.

At Christmas 1959 he went home for the first time since being admitted. His parents reported that he appeared to be very glad to be home, jumping up and down and clapping his hands. He muttered 'Dad-dad, Mum-mum, Night-night' in a sing-song fashion, playing happily without needing constant attention. He was still kept in napkins and had no ability to control his toilet habits. This progress was continued on returning to West Stowell. In March 1960 he showed the first signs of interest in toilet control and this progressed slowly throughout the year. Andrew showed great interest in nursery rhymes. Treatment consisted mainly of regressed nurtural care, with an additional concentration by the therapist on speech. As the year proceeded he seemed happier in himself, and began to hum nursery rhymes to himself. At the same time his attitude towards adults changed from clinging dependence to demanding and attention-seeking. His parents reported further improvement, both generally and in understanding, when he went home in August.

In December 1960, at 5 years old, his manual dexterity was roughly appropriate to age, but his general behaviour and emotional attitudes were those of a 2-year-old. His Christmas leave brought new improvements in most fields. By the beginning of 1961 Andrew began to develop speech, including a few words in the songs he hummed. He seemed to understand a great deal of what was going on around him, and could carry out relatively complex activities when asked to do so. He still banged his head on the floor if he did not get his own way, but such tantrums were rarer.

In April he was transferred to a play group that contained more advanced children, and here he made good progress. He liked to look at picturebooks and draw, and was able to name objects, although it was not until the end of the year that he would go beyond this to conversation with his therapist. However, he was building up a fairly extensive vocabulary, and had also learned to recite numbers up to ten by the end of the year.

His parents had noted considerable progress with speech at home. He could understand all their requests to him and was beginning to form short sentences of two or three words, at first by repetition but later using them spontaneously. He also learned to dress and undress himself, improved greatly in toilet control so that he was seldom incontinent by day in the latter part of the year, and was showing a lively interest in all around him, testing people and things, constantly exploring and extending his experience. Many of his social achievements coincided with his being placed in a small family group with a housemother and -father. Meals and bedtime now became pleasurable occasions and he seemed eager to please his houseparents by helping at these times. He also showed some awareness of the group situation and moved a little away from his previous egocentric attitudes. His houseparents found that he was soon able to produce crude but imaginative pictures which suggested that he might have talent in this sphere. He could also write his name and seemed pleased at this achievement.

By his sixth birthday, in December 1962, the management of his case continued to stress contact with the family group with the aim of bringing him closer to the appropriate social level for his age. Hence, in January 1963 Andrew started in the nursery class. Here he had more opportunity to name objects and draw without being interrupted. He started making crude drawings of aeroplanes and, gradually, after being shown pictures and models, developed a detailed and sophisticated style, producing dozens of pictures of rockets, satellites, and planes with an occasional boat or train drawn when specifically encouraged and supervised. He also made models of planes, again with a striking eye for detail. As long as he was absorbed in such activities and not being disturbed by other children he was no trouble and often seemed like a normal child of about 4, but he was still very prone to outbursts of temper and screaming if upset. Little attempt was made to direct him into formal school activities, but he was encouraged to read familiar words and could recognize several of these. He would not sit for more than ten minutes so that much of his time was spent looking at other people's work until he chose to draw again. There was little change in his egocentric attitudes, and even by the end of the year he seemed to have no concept of what the school class was for. Despite this, his teacher felt he had considerable ability and that he should eventually make good progress. His speech was developing slowly but in a rather manneristic way, with a tendency to echolalia. He usually called himself 'Andrew' rather than 'I' and 'me' but by the end of the year was showing some capacity for seeing things in 'my' and 'your' terms.

Early in 1963 Andrew was transferred to a more formal class under a trained ESN teacher. He was still mainly interested in things that attracted his attention, but he now seemed ready to deal with imposed activities. His teacher found him willing to learn and able to cope with most tasks given to him. His speech was at a level where it no longer hindered progress, and the main difficulty was to get him to accept the classroom situation and enjoy activities such as reading and writing. Alongside this progress at school, he went through a disturbed period in the house. His housemother found him suddenly very dependent on her and regressing to head-banging activities if not comforted by nursing. He also reacted excessively to other children.

In some ways this disturbed period seemed to be tied to the greater demands being made on him at school, and as he became used to his teacher and the more formal atmosphere his tension away from the classroom eased. His school work progressed very well, and all his reports were promising. By the end of the year he could write several words and read short phrases, and was starting to do sums. His main interest remained drawing, especially aeroplanes. When his houseparents left, in October 1963, after two years, his reaction was almost one of relief, as if the combined demands of school and family group had been too much for him. Andrew was now nearly 7. He had responded well to treatment and schooling, but remained so vulnerable that he seemed likely to be in the unit for at least another four years. If he advanced well, he would be able to go on to school for the educationally subnormal and hence formal education was continued even if it sometimes had a disturbing effect on him.

In September 1964 it was decided to send Andrew to the local village school for a trial period. He was proud of this and enjoyed the experience but had no idea of how to behave, and disrupted the class by constantly wandering around and talking to the other children. His speech was very stilted and concrete in its content, and this seemed possibly to be one factor in his difficulties at school. Often when asked questions he made an automatic response of 'Don't know', if he was at all uncertain of the answer. After one month the headmaster of the school asked for him to be kept at West Stowell for the rest of the term as he did not yet seem ready to accept a formal classroom situation. Andrew was very upset at this and refused to do any work in the unit's class. The period was marked by depressive and dependent attitudes rather than tempers.

At Christmas 1964 his parents found him still full of feelings of inadequacy over school and said that he had shown more tantrums and a more demanding attitude than for some years. In January 1965 he recommenced attendance at the village school and was described still as disruptive and unpredictable. Nevertheless, in the house he was now making very good progress, having a good relationship with his houseparents who, over the year, noticed a steady improvement in his capacity for speech and in his self-confidence.

At the end of the term the headmaster reported that Andrew was not without intellectual ability and academic potential, but that he was virtually impossible in a large class, as he would have a tantrum if not allowed to do what he wanted, and was constantly disturbing the other children. In fact, Andrew fared better in the summer term. His report said he possessed at least average intelligence, though this had not been translated into academic achievements because of temperamental difficulties. He displayed an above-average standard of draughtmanship in his drawing. He responded well to encouragement and was left to do work as he felt ready to, rather than being forced to work at the same pace as the other children. In this term he mixed well with other children, joining in some team games. His social and personality development were now satisfactory. Throughout this year Andrew had been having regular and successful home leaves. His parents found him less demanding and often had a whole leave without a tantrum. His toilet, dressing, and eating habits were now at an average level for his age.

New houseparents who came during the next year found him inclined to be overdependent and to regress to infantile attitudes. Also he displayed, and seemed likely to continue displaying, a lack of social awareness. This manifested itself in a number of ways. He would wander around the unit swearing loudly to himself or making

110

funny faces at people. He lacked any sense of humour, and dealt with jokes in an uncomprehending rational way – as when his house-father talked to another boy about 'selling' one of his friends and commented 'That would never do. What would we do if we sold poor old Bobby?' Andrew replied, 'Buy a tape-recorder.' There were signs of some change from his egocentric attitude in that he would bring back sweets for all his group, and ask for presents for other boys as well as himself, but for the most part life circled around himself. People were nice because they did not get cross with him, and brought him presents.

His latest major interest was with cathedrals and he drew these in preference to planes. He had collected a large number of picture postcards of them and could draw detailed representations of many from memory. At school he still had a tendency to wander, generally did what he wanted rather than what was expected, but no longer had tantrums and was less disruptive. Initial hopes for his educational attainments seemed optimistic in retrospect, but there seemed good reason to think he should be able to go home within a year or so, attend a school for the educationally subnormal and eventually hold a job of a semi-skilled nature, provided he could have a protected environment. He is likely to be an emotionally unstable and eccentric adult, but there are many attractive sides to his personality and his drawing skill seems to offer one possible avenue for development.

2. ARNOLD

Born: 20 March 1959
Admitted: 19 September 1963 for one week
Readmitted: 8 February 1965
Reason for admission: 'autistic' child, with suspected brain damage
   No speech, overactive, and withdrawn
Height: 4 ft   Weight: 3 st 3 lb

IQ: untestable
EEG no abnormality
Skull X-ray: normal, head circumference large for age
Bone-age: 6 years when 6
Treatment: regressed nurtural care in therapeutic play group; child-centred intensive care in family group

Arnold was born in a hospital in the tropics. His mother, 37 years old, had a normal pregnancy, but his birth was postmature and difficult, entailing a high forceps delivery following an artificial induction of labour. The baby weighed 8 lb 14 oz. Breast-fed for six weeks, he had to be transferred to a bottle because his mother developed a breast abscess. He appeared normal in the first weeks of life.

By his second month development was less satisfactory. He had a febrile illness from which he soon recovered, but after this was a miserable baby, crying frequently and sleeping badly. Soon after this he had a convulsion and began to bang his head against his hands. Throughout his first six months it was remarked that he was unresponsive.

Returning from home leave to Asia, Arnold was placed in the care of a nurse girl with whom he had a dependent relationship, seeing little of his mother. He began to spend much of his time sitting cross-legged and rocking from side to side, a habit which has persisted. His parents noticed that he peered at objects in a strained manner and thought he might have abnormal sight. Motor development was advanced and he was walking by the time he was 1 year old, but he continued to pay little attention to other people, living life very much on his own terms and appearing quite happy in a self-centred way.

At 15 months old his parents took him on leave, this time travelling continuously for about ten weeks. After this he became restless and destructive, and they found it hard to control his behaviour. He still showed no interest in other children, preferring to play and rock alone. At 2 years he spoke his first words saying 'Yes', 'No', and 'Up there', but his speech did not develop beyond this. At 2½ he was assessed at a London hospital for his withdrawn and unpredictable behaviour and diagnosed as autistic, separation from his nurse at 15 months being seen as a possible key factor. His parents were advised to take Arnold back to a baby regime and try to pick up

112

where his development had apparently stopped. They tried to put this into practice, but his condition showed no improvement. He had lost the little speech he had developed and now had frequent tantrums if frustrated. On the other hand, he was now toilet-trained and walked and ran well.

In 1963 Arnold's father asked for admission to West Stowell House. He was due to take up a new appointment abroad but Arnold's mother would stay in England for a few months to help him settle in at the unit. The parents explained that they had failed to get Arnold to relate to them. He was a cheerful child but had made no progress in speech or learning, was interfering and destructive, and had frequent temper tantrums. Much of his time was spent sitting alone, rocking, and if given toys he would mouth them and then threw them away.

Arnold was seen by the writer and brought to West Stowell on 19 September 1963 by his mother, who stayed for the weekend. He was a sturdy child for his age, alert, agile, and deft in manner and movement. He was very restless and detached, wandering around the consulting-room, tearing paper and emitting speech-like sounds. Placed in a family group, he settled quickly in a detached way, finding a corner where he could rock and hum to himself. He spent some hours each day with his mother, who confessed that she was upset by the presence in the unit of patients far worse than her son. On the Monday after Arnold's admission his mother decided she would take him home.

In this short period Arnold showed the signs of early infantile autism, especially when his early history was taken into account. Apart from occasional clinging, especially to his mother, he had shown little attachment to people. He was overactive physically, but not hyperkinetic. He was not actively contrary but was reluctant to pay attention to adults. He was detached and watchful, and when he gained confidence would leave his rocking to test out and cling to adults. Despite the assumption that his condition was founded on gross brain damage, no neurological indications had been found. The general impression was of a psychotic and probably sub-clinically brain-damaged child.

While abroad Arnold attended a special day school but did not learn, and his illness became worse. Overactivity and destructiveness increased, but not speech. Mental deficiency following brain damage

113

at birth began to be suspected, and after two negative EEGs a basic brain operation was advised. Meanwhile his father reapplied for admission to West Stowell, and when the child was received in February 1965, decided against brain surgery, which would have been largely experimental.

On readmission Arnold's mother brought a long list of his fads and fears, including that he hated wool next to his skin, was very frightened if clothes were pulled over his head or when his hair was washed or cut, and that he was afraid of cold or any new sensation. He was toilet-trained but needed assistance. At home he frequently received Atarax, but only if mixed with a fresh grapefruit cut up and left in its skin. He drank milk, ate bread and butter and Marmite, meat, if covered with tomato ketchup and vegetables, and had an almost obsessional fondness for ice-cream. His mother, who agreed to spend one month a year in England to help contact, was still identified with Arnold but somewhat detached in attitude.

On readmission after a very long air flight, Arnold settled well, was an alert, smiling child, sitting alone and rocking much of the time, with little overt interest in activities around him. He liked to be picked up, tickled, or swung, and seemed aware of what was going on around, although not participating. He appeared to understand much of what was said to him and would obey commands and co-operate if spoken to slowly and quietly.

He was placed in a family group that consisted mainly of rather older children. At first he only watched others, but later began to copy their actions, especially at meal and bath times, and the older children were encouraged to play with him and help him perform simple tasks. At night he received special attention, going to bed earlier than the others, and being fussed over for this additional period. This helped him to settle where previously he had woken early and occasionally soiled.

Routine care maintained toilet-control during the first month, and Arnold used the WC unaided. Fear of baths was overcome by gradual introduction and sharing with another child on a few occasions. Initial apprehension of many foods eased as he was encouraged to try small amounts with other children and he soon liked most savoury foods, if chopped up for him, whereas after admission he had been eating only milk and Complan. He could also be persuaded to eat bread and potato if Marmite were added.

114

In March his mother, who flew over to visit him, seemed more relaxed, warm, and natural in attitude to Arnold. He recognized her and showed immediate affection, and eleven days' Easter leave with her passed smoothly with only occasional temper tantrums.

Treatment in his first six months consisted largely of regressed nurtural care. At first, while in the therapeutic play group, he sat on the window ledge, rocking and humming but covertly watching everything going on. His play therapist made no attempt to break into this activity for some weeks, but greeted him frequently with a smile and the offer of a sweet, and took him to the toilet at regular intervals during the day. Initially he withdrew from her, turning away with an anxious look to another corner of the room, but after a month he would accept a sweet and ask to go to the toilet. Later still he began to accept physical contact, hand-holding and being cuddled, and after six months would occasionally approach an adult and reach out his arms to be lifted, or lead his play therapist to the swings. He manifestly enjoyed the gardens, especially climbing and playing in water. In June 1965 he had attended his first party. Before the event he seemed anticipatory, enjoying the sight of balloons and other decorations, but when it started he became anxious, and after half an hour was glad to leave and go to bed. At later parties in October and at Christmas he enjoyed the music and colour, though was content to stay on the fringe of activities.

By the end of 1965 Arnold was a much happier and more interested child, enjoying adult contact for short periods, and ceasing to rock if approached with affection. In his play group, interest in building bricks and other constructive activities developed, and a cheerful 'Arnold, pack it in!' could stop him from his rocking. A tentative relationship with a smaller child began, too, and they would romp together, laughing happily. He was still not speaking, except to say 'Wee, wee' when he wanted to go to the toilet. Toilet habits were good, and he was concerned about being clean.

Houseparents and play therapist found he responded to words but showed little interest in any verbal relationship, whereas physical contact evoked a good response. He spent time building brick castles if stroked and encouraged. He showed increasing interest in his family group and would follow what they were doing and allow them to help him. He was also encouraged to help with simple tasks like clearing the table. When his houseparents left in December

1965 he showed no signs of missing them and transferred his dependence to other members of the group.

Arnold spent a trouble-free Christmas with relatives, but was still out of contact. His mother returned to England in March 1966, and on her arrival at the unit he rushed up to her and flung his arms around her. She was strongly affected by this change in attitude and misjudged the amount of improvement made. On a fortnight's Easter holiday in rural Wales with her he was often very agitated, urinating frequently and holding his penis excessively. He also had bouts of giggling. His mother was encouraged to continue having him for short periods, usually less than a week, especially in unfamiliar surroundings. She seemed bound up emotionally with Arnold and reluctant to make a realistic appreciation of his slow progress.

By May 1966 Arnold was 7 years old. He had accepted new houseparents happily. Apart from transient frequency of micturition, his habits were normal and he was mainly conforming. He still produced little speech but seemed to understand what was said to him and occasionally silently mouthed words. Frequently he wore a lost and puzzled expression though this gave way to delight when he was able to run around in the gardens and bathe in the paddling pool. He showed little interest in constructive play activities and seemed in most respects to be making only slow progress in relationships and contact with his environment. This is in keeping with the general experience of the unit that the first year of treatment in the case of autistic children is a period of cautious observation as they evaluate the environment from the viewpoint of its threat potential.

3. BILLY

Born: 11 August 1959

Admitted: 23 March 1965

Reason for admission: Psychotic child, very overactive and destructive. Considered too disturbed for the children's unit to which he had been admitted for investigation of possible auditory imperception

Height: 3 ft 7½ in   Weight: 3 st 6 lb 7 oz

IQ: untestable

EEG: normal
Skull: X-ray normal
Bone-age: 5 years when 5
Treatment: regressed nurtural care
   therapeutic play group
   child-centred intensive care in family group

Billy was referred to West Stowell House after being seen at two hospitals. He had been excluded from nursery school and training centre because of destructive, hyperkinetic behaviour. He was relatively unsocialized and his disturbance seemed likely to have an organic underlay; the prognosis was poor.

Billy was born after a normal pregnancy and confinement. Labour was short with a precipitate second stage. He weighed 7 lb 4 oz. He sat up at 6 months, crawled at 8 months, walked at 13 months, and was feeding himself by 1 year. Breast-feeding failed after two weeks. He did not respond to toilet-training, and by 18 months had developed fear of the toilet and seemed obsessed with excretion.

At 2 he was beginning to speak, but shortly after this he began to regress and within a year lost speech and became withdrawn and aggressive. This change coincided with the birth of his sister and first showed in increased anxiety over any change of environment. After a room had been painted he persistently asked 'Where has the yellow door gone?' and became obsessional about every piece of furniture having its fixed place. He also became very bothered about the lights in a nearby factory. In addition, he withdrew into himself and would not play with other children. He became overactive, demanding, and difficult to control, especially if taken shopping, and was increasingly impulsive and unpredictable.

At 4 Billy entered school but was excluded after a few weeks as beyond control and incapable of formal education. He was still not toilet-trained and his eating habits had deteriorated. There was still occasional sporadic speech, but by now he was a manifestly abnormal child. He had developed a number of overt psychotic symptoms, climbing over objects, balancing on furniture, and jumping off it with a scream. He scooped up water from puddles or the WC, sucking it into his mouth and spitting it out in an upwards direction. At times he slapped his face violently and let out a sharp cry, especially if he was frustrated over something. He had also

117

been seen to pick at his eyes and even to poke his fingers into them, causing chronic inflammation.

He entered hospital for eight days in March 1964, after which infantile psychosis was diagnosed. During this stay he appeared oblivious of his surroundings. On discharge he had lost any speech that had remained. He then entered a training centre but was soon excluded, after jumping through the window and climbing up a fire escape.

In October 1964 he was admitted to a children's psychiatric unit and diagnosed as psychotic. During his stay he showed affectionate responses towards staff and enjoyed musical activities, but was felt to be too disturbed for the unit. He continued to be a messy eater and poor sleeper, and would only defecate onto newspaper, screaming if taken to a lavatory or placed on a pot.

The writer saw Billy at the end of 1964 and agreed to a trial admission. His condition seemed serious, and probably organic, and although the prognosis was gloomy, it was felt he might respond to regressed nurtural care. Both parents seemed concerned and interested, but defeated by the problem. They agreed to participate in his care, and have him home for regular leaves.

On admission Billy showed no emotion when his parents left, but later became very upset, crying violently, pulling at his clothing, and picking at the edge of his eye. Later he settled and ate a meal with enjoyment.

Billy at this time was 5½, a sturdy, fair-haired child with blue eyes and ruddy complexion who stood squarely like a boxer, apparently watchful and resentful of all around him. He showed little other interest in his surroundings, sitting alone much of the time, poking at his eyes, but at times drawing attention to himself by spitting and screaming. He slept badly, waking screaming, and disturbing other children. He was careless in toilet habits, frequently walking away from the lavatory before he had finished urinating.

It was noticed that he was fascinated by surfaces and textures, and that he sometimes mouthed unsuitable objects, even eating them. He was unable to dress himself, and would allow an older child or a member of staff to dress him. He did not talk at all, but there was little positive withdrawal. In the gardens he proved an agile and active child who loved to climb trees and swing.

The first few months at West Stowell brought little change. His initial depressed state proved transient, but occasional bouts of screaming continued. He still liked to spit, but this was usually not directed at a person and seemed to be partly exploratory and partly a skill-using activity. He was placed in a play group with rather more robust children, where he was able to be specially mothered. He enjoyed being nursed and it was found that he responded to simple requests.

He went home for a short Easter leave in 1965. His parents reported that he was worse in behaviour, especially in aggression towards his sister. On return to the unit he tended to revert immediately to screaming and crying when his parents visited, investigating what they had brought him but showing no interest in them as people. His toilet and eating habits remained primitive and he would grab food from the plates of other children. To help him, he was transferred to a family group containing younger children who were more withdrawn. He seemed to respond well to this, and to enjoy being managed at baby level.

In June 1965 Billy was assessed as suffering from a partially reactive infantile psychosis, as he did not now seem essentially autistic. It was felt he had probably had an underlying developmental abnormality which revealed itself in emotional vulnerability at the time of his sister's birth and resulted in his anxious, aggressive behaviour and bizarre mannerisms. His apparently self-damaging activities often seemed to be done deliberately to test adults' reactions.

By July, after four months, Billy began to show some response to treatment. He had established a good robust relationship with his play therapist, and showed considerable pleasure in being nursed and in romping with her. The possibility of being able to roam freely, climb trees, and play on the garden swings seemed to have helped him, and he showed little aggression towards other children unless provoked, when he would effectively deal with children much bigger than he was. He was easily frightened by sudden loud noises, and at such times would become rigid. He was still easily upset and would hit himself on the face in anger if frustrated. He spent two weeks at the end of July with his parents, who found him less overactive and easier to control. In the unit his spitting and eye-probing had diminished considerably, and he seemed much happier. His alert interested appearance belied his low operational level, and made final diagnosis difficult. Speech was still absent apart from monotonously repeated 'Mum–mum; Dad–dad–dad'. Over the next few months he showed some progress in his play group, attempting simple jigsaws and playing ball with his play therapist. In his family group his toilet and eating habits remained at a poor level. By the end of the year Billy, now 6, had maintained his stabler attitudes, but had made no further progress in social habits and skills. He had become more self-assertive and aggressive as he gained confidence in his surroundings and was also much more cheerful and outgoing than on admission. It was expected that he would make further progress under regressed nurtural care as he had established a good relationship with the play therapist.

At Christmas his parents found him more dependent and responsive than on admission, and remarked on his apparent interest in their company. By May 1966 Billy had made some progress in verbal contact and would say 'Yes' and 'No'. His parents still found him difficult at home, but in the unit he seemed less unstable emotionally and was much improved in eating habits. He was toilet-controlled under supervision but otherwise tended to ignore the pot and defecate on the floor or in the garden. He would stack bricks with the help of his play therapist and enjoyed playing ball and scribbling in a book, but had made no progress towards spontaneous constructive play. There were signs of continuing aggression to other children, on whom he would from time to time make unprovoked attacks. On the other hand, his approach to adults was now confident and communicative, though usually concerned with immediate needs.

4. BOBBY

Born: 21 April 1952
Admitted: 23 June 1959
Readmitted: 5 October 1961
Reason for admission: grossly disturbed behaviour at home and school, including temper tantrums, head-banging, and destructiveness. Mother had just given birth to her fifth child
Height: 3 ft 7 in   Weight: 3 st
IQ: 55 (1958)
EEG: not taken

Skull X-ray: within normal limits

Bone-age: 8 years when 9½

Treatment: 1959–1960: Regressed nurtural care in play group

1961–1966: Child-centred intensive care in family group, with attendance at nursery class, and from April 1964 in formal school class

Bobby was referred to West Stowell House by a consultant children's psychiatrist who saw him because of his retarded and disturbed behaviour. He thought his retardation was probably due to some organic traumatic condition, and that he was in need of special schooling and care.

Bobby's mother was only 17 years old at the time of his birth, and had been very upset by her pregnancy, which was neither planned nor wanted. Pregnancy and birth were both normal, though labour was prolonged, lasting 30 hours. No instruments were used; the baby weighed 6 lb 8 oz and was apparently normal. He was breast-fed for six months.

Bobby was a difficult child from birth, always crying a great deal. As a baby he became very upset whenever anyone looked into his pram, never wanted to be picked up or cuddled, and took so little notice of people that he was thought deaf. From 5 months old he began to rock and bang his head.

He did not sit up independently until 12 months, crawled at 15 months, and walked at 24, but was always bumping into things. He had a severe squint, but later attempts to correct this were frustrated by his refusal to wear glasses, which he could break by stamping on them.

At 18 months temper tantrums began. He would go rigid and scream if frustrated, banging his head against the wall. He responded badly to attempts to toilet-train him, depositing motions all over the house and reacting to correction or reproval with a tantrum.

During his early life Bobby's parents were living with his maternal grandparents. His mother, who had had a disturbed and unhappy childhood, seems to have rejected him, from resentment at having become pregnant so early. There was much squabbling between his parents, neither of whom were ready for parenthood. They also quarrelled with the grandmother, who tended to 'spoil' Bobby, picking him up and cuddling him whenever he had been corrected.

By the time he was 3 years old Bobby was not toilet-trained, and had only just begun to speak and feed himself. His tantrums were growing worse, and he was using them to gain his grandmother's sympathy.

When he was 4 Bobby's parents moved to a house of their own on a new council estate which his mother did not like, although Bobby seems to have made rather better progress at first. His grandmother visited regularly, and he always made a point of saying he felt ill, so that she would fuss over him. He told his parents he did not like them, and wanted to go to live with his grandmother. Often they would pretend that he was going off with her up to the last moment, to stop him from having a tantrum. By now his parents had realized that Bobby was backward in comparison with their neighbours' children. At 4½ his mother took him to see their doctor, who told her not to worry. At 5 Bobby started to attend an infants' school. He proved consistently difficult to handle, because of constant wetting, screaming, and bad language. Frustration produced tantrums and head-banging. If given extra attention he would calm down for a while, but this was often impossible in a large class. After a year his mother agreed to keep him at home, where he received one hour's tuition a day. He was seen by a psychiatrist who diagnosed him as being in the epileptic/hyperkinetic group of mentally retarded children, and recommended special residential care as well as special schooling.

Bad behaviour at home continued. He would not mix with other children and refused to play with toys, throwing them at his mother or breaking them up. His mother, who now had two other children, found she was pregnant again. She felt she would not be able to cope, and asked for urgent help to get Bobby away. She was an emotionally immature person, resenting growing up, identifying with adolescence, and full of feelings of rejection which she projected onto Bobby. Her husband, who was four years older than herself, could control Bobby, but only by hitting him. He worked as a lorry driver but was studying to be a salesman in his spare time, which his wife resented.

Bobby was admitted on 23 June 1959 at the age of 7. He was small for his age, an attractive boy, fair-haired and blue-eyed, with a large head and a marked squint. His manner was alert and inquisitive, but appropriate for a child some years younger.

He appeared unmoved when his mother left, accepting his new situation but showing little warmth towards staff. Speech was good, though hurriedly delivered, and he carried on sensible conversations with staff, asking about the unit and the names of other children. He was placed in an occupation group, where he showed interest in toys and some manipulative ability. During the first months Bobby was fairly subdued. His habits were clean, and he slept and ate well. As he grew accustomed to his new setting, however, his pattern of behaviour began to resemble that described by his mother at home. If reprimanded he had a tantrum or swore loudly, and if upset would tear his clothes. By October, when the writer came to West Stowell, such episodes were occurring regularly.

Bobby now began to receive regressed nurtural care in a therapeutic play group. He was happy there, and showed sufficient aptitude to be considered for the pre-school activities. As long as he was given a great deal of attention his behaviour caused no concern. However, he refused to mix much with other children, and by the end of the year had developed a marked obsession with death, going off alone and talking to himself in a sort of destructive fantasy. He talked of killing and drowning himself, and of people being hurt and killed in various ways. During early 1960 Bobby's behaviour continued fairly stable, with occasional eruptive episodes. In his play group he manipulated objects with apparent intelligence, and it was felt he would be able to cope with residential schooling at an educationally subnormal level by the end of the year, as his major problems now seemed educational in spite of his lack of educational success.

Bobby's major interest at this time was with insects and small creatures. He would put newts, lizards, and caterpillars into a box and watch them with fascination, but preferred to squash and kill insects such as flies and wasps, apparently relishing this activity. Over the year his behaviour grew more eccentric and emotional, but the violent tempers were fewer and there was less setting out to run away if rebuked. He became very dependent on one member of staff, and would run to him at the slightest provocation, clinging for reassurance in an infantile manner. He used speech freely to describe his activities, and his imagination was rich, vivid, and on a level far beyond his educational attainments.

By the end of the year, when a place was offered at a boarding school, Bobby had still made no educational progress. He was, however, discharged, since it was believed he might respond to more skilled teaching. It was also feared that he might regress in some spheres in the permissive atmosphere at West Stowell House. The most noticeable feature of his behaviour was still his aggressive, imaginative fantasy life. His talk was full of macabre references: 'Cut his throat', 'Strangle him', 'Shoot him through the head'. However, for much of the time he appeared a friendly, happy child, and when he was discharged in December it was considered there was little evidence of any severe emotional disturbance.

After two terms Bobby was excluded from the boarding school for educationally subnormal children, as he had made no progress at all and seemed quite unable to make use of what ability he had. He made no progress with reading, although he could be persuaded to repeat words when they were pointed out to him, and, with supervision, would copywrite his name in large crude letters. He had made no progress with numbers beyond parroting 'One and one makes two'. Occasional tantrums were short-lived if dealt with firmly. During the day he was toilet-controlled, but frequently wet at night. In excluding him, the headmaster said the only subject at which he showed ability was art, and suggested he needed a small group in which he could make a relationship with a teacher, after which some sort of educational progress might be possible.

On returning home in July 1961 Bobby proved as difficult to handle as ever, especially since he was at home all day, because there was no local training centre.

Bobby was readmitted to West Stowell on 5 October 1961 as being in need of further supportive therapeutic management. He was now placed straight into the school class, and into the most structured of the family groups. At school he could do nothing, was extremely noisy, and had frequent outbursts of temper, in which he would bite and smack himself if he did not get his own way. His houseparents found him a friendly boy, eager to be liked, but having little contact with other children. His toilet, eating, and washing habits were all good.

At $9\frac{1}{2}$ Bobby was still small for his age, and very retarded intellectually and emotionally. Much of the time he seemed to be living in a world of his own, and his defensive attitude towards many adults suggested that he had been intimidated in the past, or at least had never gained much assurance of adults' affection. In an attempt to overcome this, he was given intensive infantile management, while being encouraged to meet various emotional demands. Whenever he showed excessive anxiety and tension he was given special individual support by a member of staff.

His housemother left in early 1962, but Bobby did not seem unduly affected by this. By April he was 10, and the infantile nature of his behaviour was still clearer. He had made some progress, speech was improved, and he was developing an attractive sense of humour, calling himself 'Yogi Bear'. His imagination became more disorderly as he grew older, with aggressive thoughts intermingled with babyish, dependent, and hostile fantasies. In addition to his intellectual dullness, his personality disturbance now seemed more marked with several psychotic features. He was very dependent on support from adults and constantly sought attention from staff.

During 1962 his macabre fantasies, so often noted during his previous stay at West Stowell, again became apparent. He mixed very little with other children, preferring to walk in the gardens thrashing nettles with a stick and shouting 'Hang him', 'String him up'. If crossed by another child, he could become violent, throwing chairs about and usually ending in a tantrum and tears. The fascination with crawling insects and animals also persisted. His summer leave was uneventful, although his mother said he talked a lot about being hit by staff and tied down to a table, an imaginative exercise he showed more and more over the next few years, especially concerning adults who made any demands on him.

In October 1962 he was transferred from the school class to a therapeutic play group. At school his behaviour had become increasingly negativistic and turbulent. In the play group he was encouraged in pre-school activities, but was also given intensive regressed nurtural care, and treated with a tranquillizer. By the end of the year the change of treatment had not brought any major change of behaviour pattern.

Bobby spent six weeks at home at Christmas, and returned happy and noticeably plumper. A holiday report suggested that he might well have been hit frequently by his father, but he did not seem to have suffered from this. A new attempt to get him to go to school had to be dropped because of his disturbed response. In the house he seemed to be acting more and more in a psychotic manner. He was in

K

and out of touch with his environment, and his attitude towards staff swung from a threatening hostility to an infantile dependence. He had not responded to regressed nurtural care and was really too old for it now. Instead he was looked after individually by the nursing staff, spending much time with them informally and enjoying the experience. He returned to his family group for the usual family activities.

In April 1963 Bobby was 11. The next few months were marked by a mixture of depression and aggression. He went home at Easter, but felt resentful when his family went off on holiday after he had returned to West Stowell. Impulsive attacks on other children and his houseparents began. In the consulting-room he talked in a fluent striking manner, with a continuous flow of aggressive memories and ideas, many of them on a primitive level. Physically he looked like a child of 7 or 8, educationally he was at a 3- or 4-year level, yet in general social awareness, and ability to verbalize, he was only slightly retarded. The main problem seemed to be his gross lack of emotional stability and control, which led to unpredictable, damaging, and aggressive behaviour. The aim of treatment was still to ease his tension while making continuing social demands on him so that he did not slip backwards.

In the autumn Bobby was again tried at school and there were now no behaviour difficulties, although he still did not learn. Aggressive fantasies continued and he would talk to the writer of how his parents and members of staff 'bonked' him. Despite regular leaves, he continued to feel uncertain about his parents. He never knew when they would collect him for his holiday, and after receiving a letter a week for some time would suddenly receive nothing for months.

The next year, 1964, brought further slow progress. Concern with death and 'creepy' animals had waned, but he played battles with toy soldiers as if he were a 5-year-old, shouting out orders to shoot and kill. In the spring new houseparents and a new teacher came. Bobby was disturbed by this at first, but over the rest of the year showed the most constructive period of improvement since admission. At school his teacher set out to build up a good relationship with him. She also encouraged his sense of humour and so managed to avoid upsets which formerly led to inability to concentrate. His houseparents' first reaction was that Bobby was a spoilt little boy who used tantrums to get his own way, but they gradually came to realize that when he overreacted to a situation (as by running away from

126

the house after being corrected) he was really quite terrified and unable to appreciate what was going on. They tried to deal with this by ignoring his tantrums rather than attempting to placate them. After a while Bobby accepted this, and would talk later about the tantrums and what had upset him, usually providing an understandable reason. They felt a breakthrough was made with his announcement towards the end of the year that he was fed up 'with being a bloody baby'. After this his moods and tempers lessened, but he became verbally antagonistic towards his houseparents. At home he said he did not want to go back to the same family group. When another boy was taken to hospital with appendicitis Bobby said the housefather had kicked him in the stomach. For some months hostility against all members of staff continued, usually in their absence, but at the same time his behaviour at school and in his family group was maturing considerably. His appearance at 13 years was very immature, as well as being unmasculine, and there seemed likely to be an element of retarded physical development in his condition.

Bobby's progress in 1964 continued in 1965. In his family group he was helping more and taking a 'big brother' attitude towards younger members. At school he also improved although he was still over-sensitive to other children and for some time insisted on his desk touching the teacher's. Preoccupation with death and killing had disappeared, and he had developed a most unexpected interest in the Ancient Romans. This started by chance when his teacher showed him a radio schools programme pamphlet about the Roman occupation of Britain. He listened eagerly and asked for more stories, learning a number of elementary facts. His teacher made use of this near-obsessional interest to get him to try to count Roman soldiers, write the names of Roman towns, and make models of various aspects of Roman life. Over the year he produced a model villa and fortress and a detailed mosaic. Formal reading, writing, and spelling made very slow progress.

In the summer Bobby again suffered from his parents' changing their minds about when to take him on holiday but gained some compensation when a student on a study course at West Stowell became specially interested in him and took him on trips. As had been noticed before, a special relationship with one person seemed of great importance to him.

127

His teacher then left, and it was feared that Bobby would become antagonistic to school as a result, but he related quite well to her successor. His interest in Rome continued, but it was difficult to expand his interest to other things. At 13½ he could still only write and recognize his own name and no more. How much his failure to progress was due to innate intellectual dullness and how much to severe emotional disturbance was hard to decide. He could not tell the time, say what day it was, or recognize familiar words like 'Roman' and 'Hadrian's Wall'. On the other hand, he had a good spoken vocabulary and could explain fairly complex words, and relate, in a somewhat garbled fashion, several episodes from Roman history.

Bobby's houseparents left at the end of 1965, and for a time he appeared to regress in that he provoked the temporary staff and gave up helping to serve dinner and lay the table, as he had formerly. He reacted to new houseparents in March 1966 by leaving the group whenever possible, and roaming round the gardens alone or going to watch television with the domestics. When his housefather asked him to stay with them, he was at first resentful but later accepted this and became a co-operative member of the group.

He was still exceptionally vulnerable and emotionally over-labile, swinging from extreme depression and moodiness to periods of cheerful elation in which he seemed to be parodying his other moods. Other children could easily anger him by teasing. Verbal and physical attacks were met with anger and self-punishment, but he would only retaliate if supported by an adult.

By May 1966 Bobby was 14 years old. He had the physical appearance of a much younger child and remained emotionally immature. His level of play was that of a 6- or 7-year-old and still had a large element of aggression and death in it. He was very dependent on one or two adults and would hang on to these in an infantile manner, or stand around them in a dependent manner, often at a loss for words. He had found he could obtain a response from people by calling them 'Crook' and laughing, and now tended to do this all the time. He also talked about his moods, saying he was 'up the pole', and going mad, and complaining about a number of pains, bad eyesight, and so on. For most of the time he was able to cope well socially and he could get his ideas across in effective amusing language. The main problem continued to be the way in which he was

128

dominated by his moods, and especially his occasional bouts of aggression and self-punishment. He had begun to talk of being 'fed-up' with the unit and wanting to go home, but the position remained uncertain, as contact with home was irregular, although his family now seemed fond of him. It was hoped that he could go home in the next year if a suitable training centre place were found, but he might need to go on to a hostel for subnormal adolescents, where he could receive closer supervision, and more support than his home could offer.

5. CHRISTOPHER

Born: 17 August 1955
Admitted: 11 October 1962
Reason for admission: psychotic child with no speech; very disturbed emotionally
Height: 4 ft 2 in   Weight: 3 st 9 lb
IQ: 88 (scale for aphasics, 1962)
EEG: not taken
Skull: X-ray impossible to take; circumference abnormally large
Bone-age: 8 years when 8
Treatment: family-group system with child-centred intensive care
  Regressed nurtural care in a therapeutic play group

Christopher was first referred to West Stowell in September 1960 when he was attending a residential school for the deaf. He was thought to be probably psychotic, not deaf, and was later diagnosed as 'autistic'. He then went to a special hospital unit for deaf children, from which a request for admission to West Stowell was made, as he was thought to need psychiatric treatment. He was admitted to West Stowell in October 1962.

Christopher was the first child of intelligent artistic parents. His mother, who was 24 years old at his birth, had a normal pregnancy, although she recalled that in the third month she might have had a mild attack of influenza. He was a planned and wanted child. His birth was two weeks postmature and had to be induced. Labour took twenty-four hours but no instruments were used. He weighed 8 lb

8 oz and had a large head but was not thought to be hydrocephalic. His mother says that he was 'a wonderful, nice-looking boy, pink and white, not red like the others'.

Christopher was a quiet placid baby who was breast-fed for eight weeks. In his early months he seemed to take a keen interest in everything around him. Later he became more passive and disinterested. His mother said that he had always been self-sufficient and that, though given much affection, had never demanded it. He never played with cuddly toys, but liked a wooden rabbit whose ears he could manipulate.

By the time he was 12 months old, his parents were worried by his slow development. He did not sit until a year, and then with difficulty. He did not walk until 2 and showed no response to toilet-training. He did not feed himself until $3\frac{1}{2}$, and at 1 year old it was also noticed that he did not respond to sound, so that his parents thought he might be deaf. By 2 years it was clear that Christopher was not only retarded but behaved abnormally. He lived in a world of his own, wandering about carrying with him a small perspex tile or a spectacle lens. When cross he would drag his feet and bite his hands, but never cried with pain on doing this. He used adults' hands to open doors. Much of the time he sat alone, rocking or playing with bits of glass and lenses which fascinated him and which he manipulated with some dexterity. He paid no attention to other people, though his mother said that when bathed with his sister for the first time he was interested in her lack of penis.

From the age of 18 months Christopher was subjected to a series of investigations that produced conflicting diagnoses; that he was a late developer of poor intelligence, that he was of high intelligence but deaf, that he was both deaf and defective. Tests for phenyl-ketonuria had proved negative. Finally a consultant otologist recommended him to a nursery boarding school for the deaf and he went there at the age of $3\frac{1}{2}$.

In June 1960, when nearly 5, Christopher was referred to Child Guidance, where it was thought that he had 'the typical behaviour and appearance of an autistic schizophrenic'. It was impossible to make any personal contact with him, as most of the time he wandered round with a skipping gait, singing to himself, and holding a piece of coloured perspex. He showed no concern or interest when taken from his mother. He responded to simple commands, and was able to hear a watch ticking in closed hands, so serious hearing loss seemed unlikely. Diagnosis was psychosis, probably of organic basis, and aphasia, and Christopher was recommended for treatment in a special unit for psychotic children, although at the time he was said to be doing quite well at his nursery school.

In September 1960 he was referred to West Stowell House and seen by the writer. His parents recounted his history, mentioning that he was fascinated by the texture of surfaces, particularly those that were smooth and shining, and also liked to sniff at objects. He had been attending boarding school for the deaf for five terms and his parents wondered whether his self-contained and detached way of dealing with his environment might be partly due to this, as he was always glad to be brought home for the holidays.

Following a good deal of further investigation, the final assessment was that his failure to speak was probably due to an abnormal psychological state, rather than true aphasia, whether organic or developmental. Speech therapy seemed impossible, because of his lack of co-operation, and he was diagnosed as a 'pre-psychotic' child, and recommended for a school for maladjusted children.

This recommendation was not acted upon, and Christopher returned to his deaf school until the end of the year, when he was referred to a newly opened unit for deaf and aphasic children. After investigation there it was thought that Christopher was an autistic child with some underlying cerebral lesion causing his aphasia. His intelligence had been assessed as 88 on a non-verbal scale for aphasic children, and it was thought that he should be treated as severely disturbed rather than subnormal. It was, however, impossible to get him to respond to group teaching, and again psychiatric treatment was considered. In early 1962 a request for admission to West Stowell House was made and it was agreed to take him later in the year.

Christopher was brought to West Stowell by his parents. Family history revealed that an uncle had had a severe mental illness at the age of 19, and had done no work since, and an aunt was said to have had a major nervous breakdown. Mother seemed to feel that father was rather too dreamy and that he did not play a full part in family life. She had married at 21 and had had three miscarriages before Christopher. She gave the impression of having managed him in a rather over-anxious manner in his early years, when father had contracted out of any responsibility for bringing up the child.

In his first weeks at West Stowell Christopher showed no interest in his new surroundings and remained indifferent to staff approaches. There were occasional bouts of screaming and overactivity, but for the most part he was restless and detached. He made only fleeting relationships with other children. He had a number of minor food fads. Toilet habits were fairly good, but he needed dressing and undressing, and was often noisy and overactive before settling down to sleep. In his play group he showed no interest in toys or jigsaws, preferring to sit on his own, pulverizing pieces of chalk with his fingernails and then flicking the dust. He also liked to wave strips of paper and watch them flap, and to flick idly through picture books. He would carry on these activities for hours, interspersed with agitated walking to and fro flapping his hands and arms.

Treatment was planned to be mainly regressed nurtural care, and aimed at establishing some sort of human relationship at however primitive a level. This was combined with home leaves, and regular visits from his parents.

After three months Christopher showed no signs of regression, apart from occasional returns to biting himself when frustrated. On the other hand, he showed no indication of coming into contact or of developing speech. He would sometimes nuzzle up to his play therapist for physical embrace but these overtures lacked substance. He showed much delight in the loud music at the physical exercise sessions with the remedial gymnast.

At the beginning of 1963 his houseparents were helped in making special efforts to get him to join in group activities, and find some satisfaction in his surroundings. It was thought that Christopher had suffered from such a long period in boarding school at so young an age, aggravating his underlying condition, which was probably organic. It seemed essential to salvage something of his emotions as soon as possible. However, despite intensive approaches, he remained out of touch, flapping a piece of old bandage in front of his eyes, apparently gaining much satisfaction from watching this.

In February he suddenly developed a great fear of bathing, and screamed if taken near the bath. This was overcome by making bathtime into a special game, and encouraging him to play with the water and look on the bath as a pleasurable activity. He responded to this approach but hopes that bathtime routine might help in establishing a relationship were disappointed.

For the rest of the year Christopher remained detached but apparently content. There were no signs of speech or constructive play developing. A number of staff recorded the impression that, though apparently disinterested, Christopher was watching them all the time. By the end of the year he was able to dress himself, but this was done slowly and automatically. He had developed the habit of standing in a fixed posture, rocking back from right to left foot and gazing fixedly at the ceiling. This, and strip-waving, occupied much of his day despite the attempts of staff to involve him in other activities.

One promising sign was his relative success on home leaves. His reactions to these varied from a confused interest in them to an attitude of ignoring stimulation, and he usually returned without any concern. Nevertheless his parents found him much better than he had been before admission, and said that at times he seemed to be suddenly interested in what was going on and would want to help. They had no trouble with tantrums or screaming bouts as had occurred before.

Although slowly responding to regressed nurtural care, it seemed likely to be a long time before Christopher would be ready to undergo any type of education. For the first six months of 1964 he seemed more or less static, though he was slightly stimulated by the arrival of new houseparents in May. He could be stimulated into repeating a few words in a quiet rather badly articulated way, and had been heard to say the names of two play therapists.

When he returned from his summer leave he seemed to have regressed slightly. He was overactive, and more anxious and obsessional. He had been very disturbed, banging his head and hitting his face frequently, had turned out drawers and scattered powder all over the house. This followed a period in which it was thought that he was stabilizing, and when his play therapist had found a more affectionate approach to her. On one trip out with his parents he had seen an accident and exclaimed 'Oh my goodness!' the longest phrase ever heard from him.

Christopher was now 9½ It was thought he would probably need to stay at West Stowell until he was 12 or 13, after which he might be able to go home and attend a junior training centre. He had not responded to treatment as well as had been hoped, and it now seemed certain that his autistic state was organically based.

133

By the time Christopher was 10, in August 1965, his lack of further progress began to cause concern and it was thought it might be better to find him a hospital place nearer home. On the other hand, his toilet and eating habits were greatly improved, bed-wetting had stopped, and he now dressed and undressed himself. He also seemed generally happy in his solitary play, and had occasional periods of near-euphoria. At the unit party held in October he showed great interest in all that was going on and danced round dreamily but with apparent enjoyment.

In November staff changes occurred and the routine of his family group was upset. Christopher did not show any initial reaction, but his parents found him very disturbed at Christmas. He hit himself in the face, refused to dress or undress, and was frequently incontinent. The face-hitting became so bad that a course of chlorpromazine was started in an attempt to calm him down.

On returning to the unit in January 1966 Christopher was still very disturbed. His face was swollen and bruised, and he often sat screaming and hitting himself until an adult calmed him and gave him some bandage to wave. He also refused to eat, and was found to have lost nearly 3 lb in weight in a few months. To counter this, he was given a high calory, high protein diet and a period of intensive personal care. By the end of February he had regained much of his lost weight and stopped hitting himself, but had now taken to walking round with his hands clasped behind his back. He was unwilling to move them to eat, and was fed during this time. His favourite activity of strip-waving was also carried out in this position. The habit persisted even after he had become much happier in himself, and at the end of April 1966 he still wandered round the house with balletic movements, his hands clasped firmly behind him and a lost disinterested look on his face. In spite of the development of the new symptoms described above, their appearance has not been as persistent as earlier ones. He could be stimulated into using his arms, and would feed himself if sufficient care were shown.

Overall, Christopher continued as a psychotic severely subnormal boy who was moving forward developmentally only at a retarded maturational rate. The outlook was poor and his severe subnormality was likely to present as major a problem as his accompanying psychotic state.

6. DENIS

Born: 26 April 1949

Admitted: 27 February 1958

Reason for admission: juvenile psychosis; very overactive, excluded from school. Parents said they could cope but felt he needed treatment.

Height: 3 ft 10 in   Weight: 3 st 4½ lb

IQ: 29 (Merrill-Palmer 'L', March 1961)

EEG: outside normal limits – no specific epileptic or focal features

Skull X-ray: within normal limits

Bone-age: 10 years when 11½

Treatment ⎰1959: regressed nurtural care in play group for 18
Time gap ⎥ months
is more ⎨ School class for 18 months
than 18 ⎥ August 1961 onwards: family group with child-
months ⎱ centred intensive care

On admission Denis was nearly 9 years old, and had been diagnosed as mentally defective at 11 months. He had been hospitalized for much of his first two years with pulmonary tuberculosis. In recent years he had been excluded from both school and training centre because of his behaviour. His mother had a normal pregnancy, and the birth was easy. Denis was her second child. He weighed 7 lb 6 oz and appeared a normal healthy baby. Early feeding was difficult, with frequent small vomits during the neo-natal period, but these had stopped by one month. His mother was aged 27, his father 23.

He was said to develop well until he had bronchitis at 6 months old, which persisted. At 11 months he was unable to sit up without support, and was showing no outgoing interest in his surroundings. He began to lose weight, and so was admitted to hospital for observation. Diagnosis was a primary tubercular complex, but it was also thought that he was grossly defective mentally and this seemed his main problem. He made no contact with other people, showed no signs of emotion, and could not hold a spoon or cup. Although not really in need of a sanatorium bed, he was admitted because of bad home conditions.

Denis was in the sanatorium from May until October 1950. On

135

discharge his parents found him changed. He did not appear to recognize them, and no longer liked to be cuddled.

Soon after, Denis was again admitted to hospital, this time with otitis media. He stayed for several days and was thought to be suffering from some hearing impairment. At home his behaviour seems to have been abnormal. He would laugh at nothing and develop sudden irrational fears, especially at sudden noises. He was fascinated by electrical appliances, and loved to play with them.

By the age of 4 Denis was able to talk a little and in April 1953 started at nursery school. At 5 he was retained for a further twelve months, as he was not considered capable of progressing to infants' school. In May 1955 he was assessed as ineducable and placed in an occupation centre. While at the nursery school he had seemed happy and caused no trouble, though making very little progress.

Denis attended the occupation centre for two years, and then was excluded because of obscene language, and behaviour. He was aggressive towards the other children and his teacher, kicking and spitting, especially when bored or frustrated. He showed only transient interest in people, and seemed incapable of attending to anything for long. While at the centre the supervisor thought him psychotic. At 8 his social and educational achievements were still few and speech very backward. A children's consultant considered his retardation largely emotionally conditioned, and suggested hospital treatment. At home Denis seemed to have been slightly less disturbed, but his parents always minimized his oddness, and refused to admit how ill he was, stressing his lovable nature and describing him as 'stubborn but obedient'. His main pleasure at home lay in dismantling mechanical objects such as clocks.

Denis's father was described as the dominant partner in the marriage, an extravert, who was very fond of Denis and seemed able to get some response from him. The mother was more tense and anxious and a less outgoing person than her husband. Both parents failed to recognize the extent of Denis's abnormality. They considered he had a good sense of humour, which was found to mean that he was often laughing for no apparent reason. Continuing to stress Denis's good behaviour, they insisted that they only wanted him to go into hospital if it would make him better. He was admitted to West Stowell in February 1958.

Denis was then nearly 9, small and underweight for his age, but generally healthy. He approached strangers easily but with little sign of affection or interest. Speech was inadequate, containing some baby talk and 'jargon words', but a fairly extensive vocabulary. He would not answer questions about himself, and his thought processes seemed disjointed. He settled quite happily, but had little contact with his environment, and although he conformed with the other children and watched television, he made no attempt to converse with anyone. His toilet habits were poor and he was unable to wash or dress himself.

From the start Denis appeared to be living in a world of his own. He was overactive, laughing and crying without reason, and swearing frequently. His only sustained interest seemed to be in inanimate objects such as lamps and clocks, which he handled with apparent intelligence. During the first year he made no noticeable progress. His appetite improved and he lost his fear of baths. He learned to count up to five and could begin the alphabet, with the addition of an odd swear word, every few letters. There was some response to simple commands, but in general he was still detached and withdrawn, uninterested in his surroundings and other people.

In 1959 the psychotic pattern of Denis's behaviour became even more clear. His actions were repetitive and he wandered about in a dreamy absentminded manner, appearing at times to suffer from auditory hallucinations. His voice was flattish in tone, but clear and lilting. Speech was bizarre with a tendency to echolalia. As before he was fascinated by lamps, telephones, and mechanical objects. There were times when he was more in touch, and he was then less inclined to rush round hitting other children.

In October 1959 Denis was assessed by the writer as a juvenile schizophrenic. He frequently showed excessive emotional response resulting in a continuous state of heightened tension. As an immediate measure he was given chlorpromazine to help ease his tension and drive. Active treatment, concentrating on establishing relationships in a supportive environment, was started. Psychotherapeutic sessions were also given.

During the first part of 1960 Denis was treated with phenobarbitone, epanutin, and fentazin, but with little success, and after a time all medication was stopped except treatment for anaemia. In his regular sessions with the writer Denis spent much of his time investigating lamps, telephone, or light switch, while occasionally calling out 'shit', 'bugger', or 'knickers'. On one occasion he remarked, 'You are a bloody fool, Dr Kahan.'

Another aspect of Denis's condition was his continued apparent hallucinations. In the consulting-room he would suddenly say 'What did you say?' looking into a corner of the room when no words had been spoken. He had often commented on hearing music in his ears. He would wander into the nursing office and ask to see the cook but, when taken to the kitchen, would wander round, ignoring her and apparently responding to voices. A new concern was thunder and lightning, and he asked persistent anxious questions about these. On one occasion in the consulting-room he was playing with the lights in his normal fashion when he suddenly gazed at the lamp, as if deluded, and said, 'It's a house on fire.' For the rest of the session he kept talking about fire and lightning, switching the lamp on and off in apparent imitation of the latter.

On another occasion he tried to break off the heads of toy soldiers, muttering 'Poor soldiers heads off.' Once or twice he cried out, as if from a fantasy world of his own, 'Mum's dead, Denis is dead.' At moments of apparent hallucination he often bit himself, bringing up large bruises on his arms.

Denis continued to be emotionally and intellectually disorganized much of the time. He was quite incapable of dealing with the normal frustrations of a child's life and reacted excessively to many situations. His condition was manifestly psychotic, and some aspects of it suggested an organic basis. Socially he had improved very little. He still ignored toilet calls, although he had started to feed himself. He was placed in a therapeutic play group, as he had been doing nothing in the school class where he had been previously, but even in this more supportive setting he showed little response. Nevertheless, his parents were encouraged to have him for holidays at home, and he often seemed to behave better during these. His mother commented that he never wet his bed if sleeping with her!

In April 1961 Denis was 12 years old. He had been depressed and unhappy on return from his Christmas leave and, though he soon recovered, talked a great deal of his next leave at Easter. He still wetted his bed at night if not roused, and other symptoms did not lessen. His latest mannerism was to put his thumb in his mouth and suck hard at it, while wiggling his little finger. On one occasion when doing this he remarked, 'Look at Denis's windscreen wiper.' This

138

habit of referring to himself in the third person still persisted, as did his obscenities. In the consulting-room he sang a hymn tune with the new words 'Denis has shit himself'. His obscenities mingled with a newly aroused sexual awareness. He would shout 'Pants, knickers, ladies' knickers, shitty pants'. In his group he showed interest in a girl patient, saying 'Show me your cunt' and 'Rub my prick'. It was noticed that much of his drawing was of phallic symbols, especially lighthouses. He also talked of these, saying 'Johnny got killed by the lighthouse'. He was known to have had sex play with another boy patient a few years older than himself.

Home leave in summer 1961 was good, apart from one incident of setting fire to curtains. On return from this he was placed in a family-group setting, the system having just started full operation at West Stowell House. Denis showed little response to this change, and his houseparents found him distant and lacking in affection. At meals he rather dominated the situation, eating far too much, but at the same time being very faddy. An attempt to assess his intelligence level gave a score of 29 on the Merrill-Palmer 'L' scale, but this seemed totally irrelevant in view of the grossness of his mental disturbance. At times he showed flashes of intellectual ability which were well above the subnormal level. He was showing little response to treatment, and his condition, which seemed organic, remained largely unchanged, by the end of 1961.

This general pattern was continued in the first part of 1962. Sex interest was increasing, and he exposed himself to older girls once or twice. He was transferred to the more formal school class to see if he would respond better to such a situation, but the only signs of improvement were when he was at home. In view of this, it was decided that he should be sent home on a trial basis, with attendance at a training centre. If this failed, he could be readmitted to Pewsey Subnormality Hospital, in the adolescent unit.

After a number of trial leaves he went home in October 1962 and started attendance at the local junior training centre. After a fortnight he was excluded for difficult behaviour. Institutional care was recommended, but his parents said they would rather keep him at home.

On follow-up, in April 1966, when Denis was 17, he was found to be still at home, having recently commenced attendance at a new adult training centre, where he was making progress and mixing

139

well with the other trainees. He was busily engaged with contract work, which the centre was carrying out for a local firm. At home he was still self-centred and excitable, often laughing inappropriately at what was said to him. The family doctor was giving medication, and Denis was presenting domestic and neighbourhood problems. He was showing a pattern of abnormality similar to that observed at West Stowell House, but it was kept within socially acceptable limits.

7. GEOFFREY

Born: 14 March 1956

Admitted: 23 March 1964

Reason for admission: referred from a children's auditory unit as a psychotic child in need of long-term therapy and care

Height: 4 ft   Weight 4 st 4 lb

IQ: 94 (Drever Collins Junior Scale, 1963)

EEG: 1963 – sound response more in left than right temporal region

Skull X-ray: normal; circumference large for age

Bone-age: 9–10 years when aged 8

Treatment: Regressed nurtural care in therapeutic play group

Child-centred intensive care in family group

Geoffrey was referred to West Stowell from the children's auditory unit at a psychiatric hospital where he had been for two years. Diagnosis was psychosis of a non-autistic variety. He was disturbed and obsessional, having been backward since birth. Several investigations for deafness were inconclusive.

Geoffrey was two months premature and weighed 4 lb 3 oz. His mother, aged 34, vomited during pregnancy, and had an ante-partum haemorrhage at seven months, following which labour was induced. Labour and birth were easy, and Geoffrey spent five weeks in an incubator, after which he was discharged.

During his first year he showed little response to his parents and was described by his mother as a sleepy baby. When he first moved his body he lay with his head back as if he had paralysis of the neck. His parents thought him deaf. He was bottle-fed until 2 years old because he refused solids, seeming unable to swallow. He never crawled but wriggled around on his stomach and did not sit until he was 15 months old. He walked at 2 years and was slow in responding to toilet-training.

In 1958 Geoffrey was admitted to a children's hospital for suspected deafness. On return home, after three weeks' investigation, his parents claimed he was different. He could no longer walk, and had slipped back in several other directions. He was very cowed, and spent much time sitting withdrawn on the floor, flicking the pages of a book. The only interest he showed was in going for a walk or being bathed. When put to bed he would hold himself rigid, his hands stiff under the bedclothes. After his parents had left the room he would take his hands out and relax, but if they looked in later he again shot his hands under the blankets, in apparent terror.

He had been diagnosed as being deaf and grossly retarded. Skull X-ray, urine tests, etc., revealed no specific abnormality, but it was thought that his disabilities predisposed him to an overdependence on others and a lack of social contact. During his time in hospital he seems to have been subjected to a battery of tests, but no attempt at treatment was reported.

Geoffrey spent the next year at home, and at the end of 1959 was seen at an ear, nose, and throat hospital. Tested on the Merrill-Palmer scale he was found dull to average on non-verbal items, but it was noted that he was very retarded in his personal and social development.

He was easily frustrated and very self-willed. After further tests on his hearing it was considered that he was probably not deaf, but brain-damaged or suffering from a severe emotional disturbance. His parents were told to report back every six months.

In February 1962 he was admitted to hospital for further investigations, and treatment this time. A recent intelligence assessment had been 95 on the Merrill-Palmer scale and it was felt he needed treatment as a disturbed child who was probably deaf or aphasic. In fact he proved difficult to teach because of his poor concentration. He continued to be without speech and his movements were noticed to be awkward and fumbling. In view of this he was moved to an annexe of the hospital where he would have a more normal home environment, as he seemed to be very disturbed emotionally, apart from any sensory deprivation. He was tried at school, but was not able to play any part in group activities and needed a great deal of attention

L

141

before he would co-operate. He was able to match words and do difficult jigsaws, and seemed to have some concept of size, order, and number.

By July 1963 it was clear that Geoffrey was in need of long-term intensive therapy, and it seemed undesirable for him to go home in view of his parents' emotional instability. A request was, therefore, made for a place at West Stowell. He was admitted four months later, in March 1964. Probable diagnosis was juvenile psychosis of chaotic type, possibly with organic underlay.

Geoffrey's mother was an intelligent woman, who said she had not found him an easy child to handle. She had been opposed to him going to hospital and took some time to become realistic about his problems. His father was an anxious, neurotic man, once described by a visiting social worker as a 'paranoid and depressive psychopath', and he certainly seems to have been very unstable.

Geoffrey had spent three months at home before coming to West Stowell. During this time he was impulsive and unpredictable and required constant supervision, although he would play with familiar toys in a repetitive way. His grandmother, who lived nearby, helped by taking him for walks, which he enjoyed.

On admission at 8 years he could dress and undress himself, manage his own toilet, and was well-behaved at table. However, he needed constant attention and supervision. He liked to turn on taps and would throw toys around and also plates and cups if not kept under constant observation. At mealtimes he was generally conformative but faddy, liking fried food and milk, but refusing to eat bread and butter or drink tea. He ignored other children, refused to join in any group activities, and dealt with adult intervention by turning away and running off. When upset or frustrated he screamed, and would become angry if even mild pressure were applied to him.

Geoffrey was placed in a therapeutic play group, where a number of mannerisms were noted. He liked to spin toys and to lets and fall through his fingers into the sand tray, watching it flow, with obvious satisfaction. His favourite activity was to tear up paper and 'post' it through cracks in the floor or a chair. In the garden he would poke a hole to provide openings to 'post' stones and twigs. All these activities were carried out with great absorption, and he became very upset if they were interrupted.

Over the next few months it became clear that Geoffrey was a very nervous and anxious child. At times he appeared completely deaf, but responded belatedly to some requests, which seemed to indicate elective hearing. He still tried to avoid contact with adults, and became very upset if he were taken out of a setting, shrieking and hitting his face with his fist. It was decided to treat him by means of regressed nurtural care, to establish a relationship with his play therapist. This happened by slow stages. First he would approach only to take sweets, but later began to derive pleasure from physical contact and early on would take his therapist's ear in his mouth, which she accepted as a useful contact which could be developed. At the same time, much of Geoffrey's anxiety diminished, and he became more relaxed and cheerful. In his family group, too, he began to show a greater confidence in adults. He rolled round the unit with a peculiar and awkward gait, very pigeon-toed and with an apparent inversion from his hips, but was quite agile in climbing trees, and did not appear unduly hampered by these motor abnormalities.

Geoffrey was visited regularly by his mother, and in August 1964 went home on his first leave, which his parents felt showed an improved stability and fewer outbursts of temper. His father constantly asked when he would start school and how long it would be before he got better.

In the unit Geoffrey was slowly becoming relaxed and outgoing. He made friendly, smiling overtures to staff and children, often rather upsetting the latter by putting his arms around them. He still tended to do all this without looking at the person concerned and he made no attempt to communicate by language. In his family group he had a rudimentary play-relationship with Andrew, a boy of his own age and syndrome; in his play group he was showing some ability in arranging coloured blocks, but still preferred to push toys and paper down holes and crevices.

After six months further limited progress was made. At times his staggering gait and apparent deafness made his condition seem essentially an organic one, yet there were elements which required interpretation in terms of gross emotional disturbance. Whatever its origin, he seemed to be suffering from a mental disorder of psychotic intensity which had persisted since early childhood. A working hypothesis was that he had a vulnerable personality, aggravated by physical and environmental factors.

By the beginning of 1965 Geoffrey was less anxious and aggressive, but still out of contact. He had enjoyed the Christmas party at the unit, albeit in a detached way. On return to West Stowell, after his Christmas holiday, he was wetting several times daily, though leave was said to have been quite successful. His general behaviour pattern continued largely unchanged. He screamed when frustrated, clambered over furniture and people alike, but with more awareness, and spent a little less of his time 'posting' objects. In his family group he maintained a fair level of social capacity with improved mood- and self-control.

During the rest of the year Geoffrey's parents continued to visit regularly and he went home for leaves. These seemed neither to stimulate nor upset him. His general behaviour pattern showed little change. Speech did not progress, and it seemed likely that he had at least moderate hearing loss. His walking was unusual in several respects. He rarely walked straight, preferring to spin or to move sideways with a determined stamping of one foot. He liked to jump around his playroom, and to leap off tables in a noisy fashion. However, he would now approach any adult who came to the group, gazing up at them happily with his head leaning to one side, and liked to be held while he did a backward somersault. He played in a rough but unaggressive manner with one or two of the other children. If stopped from any action or requested to give up a toy taken from another child, he often reacted by screaming and kicking the wall, but such bouts were short-lived and seemed largely habit. He still spent much of his time face down on the floor, determinedly 'posting' any suitable objects into the cracks between floorboards, and his obsessive interest and pleasure in this activity showed no signs of lessening. It was hard to distract him or to get him to undertake any new form of play. By the end of the year he was considered to be more affectionate and less anxious, but to be only slightly less overactive and detached.

By May 1966 Geoffrey was 10 and had been at West Stowell two years. His symptoms were similar to those described at the end of 1965. He was very cheerful most of the time, and soon got over frustrations. On a few isolated occasions he had been observed to scream and stamp for no apparent reason, almost as if hallucinated, but these moments soon passed. In the consulting-room he responded definitely to simple requests and commands, though only after an interval. His play therapist reported occasional response to spoken words, though she found gesture more effective. He remained an isolated child and still spent most of his time on posting activities, running out of his play group to find paper if none was available there. If encouraged and supervised by his play therapist, he would build bricks with some skill and do jigsaws, but he was far from ready to enter even a nursery-school class. His gait was still clumsy, but seemed to have improved slightly since admission. He was, however, operating at a very retarded level in all spheres and had at no stage shown the potential suggested by the early intelligence tests.

8. GLYN

Born: 9 August 1955
Admitted: 14 December 1961
Reason for admission: spiteful aggressive behaviour towards other children; toilet obsessions, bed-stripping, and destructiveness at home; disruptive behaviour and gross retardation at school
Height: 4 ft 1½ in   Weight: 3 st 6½ lb
IQ: 38 (Terman-Merrill 'L', 1962)
EEG: normal
Skull: moderate degree of brachycephaly; otherwise no abnormality
Bone-age: 7 years when 7
Treatment: Child-centred intensive care in family group
   1962–1965 (Sept.): regressed nurtural care in therapeutic play group with three unsuccessful attempts at schooling
   September 1965–1966: nursery/Froebel class with periods of regressed nurtural care when necessary

Glyn was referred by his local authority because of continued disturbed behaviour following exclusion from school. Recent investigation had suggested that he was likely to have a form of childhood psychosis.

Glyn's mother, at 33, had had an easy pregnancy, and his birth, though prolonged, was normal. Glyn was her only child. He weighed 7 lb 3½ oz at birth and was bottle-fed for nine months. His parents said he was always very quiet, too good a baby. He sat up at 8 months, did not crawl but pulled himself along by 10 months and was standing at 14 months. He did not walk freely until he was 20 months old. He was very slow in other respects, being nearly 4 years old before he said even a few words, or showed any response to toilet-training. From about this time he became increasingly over-active and aggressive, especially towards younger children. He was very resistant to continuing toilet-training, kicking and screaming if taken to a lavatory, and for some time defecating only onto news-paper.

In June 1958 Glyn spent two weeks in hospital for investigation. During this time he is said to have been strapped to his bed and under almost continuous sedation. Diagnosis was simple oligophrenia, and it was stated that there was 'no evidence of raised intracranial pres-sure to account for his occult hydrocephalus'.

On returning home his behaviour had worsened. Over the next two years he became very aggressive to other children and on occa-sions towards his mother. At the end of this time he was beginning to talk, but speech was babyish and repetitive. He became obsessional about the lavatory, still defecating only onto newspaper, and fre-quently wetting his bed. He refused to sleep in his own bed, con-stantly trying to get into bed with his parents. They often relented and let him sleep between them.

By the time he was 5 he was quite beyond their control, and in July 1960 was admitted to a children's psychiatric hospital for obser-vation and treatment. He remained there for nearly five months. During this period he was overactive, demanding, and spiteful. Speech was highly repetitive, taking the form of 'Glyn do this; Glyn do that'. Attacks on children seemed deliberate. Afterwards he would watch their reactions and expect, and apparently enjoy, any conse-quent punishment. He did not appear to be backward mentally or physically, but his aggressive behaviour prevented attempts to teach him in a class. His language was limited, but he did not seem to have any difficulty in understanding what was said to him. On discharge it was suggested he might prove suitable for a training centre.

Early in 1961 Glyn entered nursery class at a local primary school, but was excluded after a week, as he completely disrupted the work of his class. He then went to the junior training centre, where he fitted in more easily and was taught to count up to three and to copy a few letters. Speech improved, and at home he stopped wetting.

However, towards the middle of the year his behaviour worsened again. He began deliberately knocking crockery off the table, laughing at what he had done, and watching for his parents' reaction. At the training centre he began to soil, at one stage passing a motion in his pants every day. Most nights he stripped his bed frenziedly before lying down to sleep. This seemed directed towards getting his parents to take him into their bed. They would punish him by rejection and smacking, but he paid no attention to any form of correction. His mother found his behaviour so worrying that she took him with her wherever she went, including toilet and bathroom. Many of Glyn's obsessions seem likely to have been aggravated by this intimacy, which seems to have led also to an early sexual awareness. Glyn's father had had a nervous breakdown after the war and was a voluntary patient in a mental hospital for a time. His mother had always been in indifferent health too. She suffered from peptic ulceration, which grew worse after Glyn's birth. She also complained of claustrophobia.

Glyn was admitted to West Stowell House in late 1961 at 6 years old. Although apparently unmoved by the departure of his parents, he showed distress after they had gone, and by evening was very agitated, weeping and screaming. When seen by the writer he appeared very apprehensive and asked whether this was his new school. He also asked persistently whether he would be smacked if he wet his pants. The impression given was of a psychotic child with an impulsive chaotic type of disturbance. In the consulting-room he would scatter sand, swear, or deliberately wet himself as if testing out the writer's reactions.

Glyn talked obsessively about toilet matters and appeared to be frightened of sitting on the lavatory, but he was fairly well toilet-controlled. He was most disturbed at mealtimes, refusing to eat off a plate and scattering food around the room or impulsively smashing crockery on the floor. His houseparents found him aggressive towards themselves and the other children, poking at their eyes with his fingers. He showed a slightly easier attitude to male compared with female staff.

Over the next few months Glyn's behaviour pattern became clearer. Many acts appeared deliberate and provocative; he seemed to expect some form of physical retaliation and to gain satisfaction from it. He was preoccupied with his own tense train of thought, which led to confused and complicated questions to which there appeared no

147

answer that satisfied him. His questions were particularly concerned with wetting and soiling, punishment, and when various members of staff would be on duty. Toilet obsession continued and he preferred to use the tots' miniature toilet whenever possible. On one occasion, when offered a baby's bottle, he sucked happily from it for a time, but afterwards insisted that he was really 'a big boy'.

His parents visited regularly, and Glyn was usually very clinging towards his mother. Once, when they took him to a café, he impulsively smashed a cup, but was very contrite afterwards. At Easter he went home for two weeks. He was very excitable but did not wet his bed or smash any crockery. His mother reported that he frequently tried to poke at her eyes with his fingers and seemed to be asking obsessive questions all the time. He was very demanding of her attention and would tear his clothes or mess his pants if he did not get it.

Much of Glyn's symptomatic behaviour, his obsessional interest in excretion, his habit of clawing at eyes, his concern with death, injury, and punishment, seemed to spring from the conflict between having been pressed to give up his infantile situation, and his deep conscious or unconscious desire to remain at a level of omnipotent infantility. It was decided to treat him by means of regressed nurtural care, giving him opportunities to work and act out his infantile yearnings. At his previous hospital it had been noted that he was happiest when playing with water and sand.

Towards the middle of the year Glyn showed more aggression towards other children, but this seemed to result from disturbance arising from staff changes. On August leave his parents found him easier to get on with. They took him to the seaside, where he enjoyed paddling and playing with sand, and the only respect in which they found him worse was that he had developed a habit of swearing loudly in public.

In the autumn new houseparents at first found Glyn very disturbed, attacking other children and scratching himself severely. He constantly asked questions such as: 'Are you going away?', 'When will you go for good?', 'Will you go to hospital?' Later he became obsessive about whether his housefather would punish him if he did certain things. He frequently passed motions in his pants and pushed his fingers down his throat until he choked. While at home for a week in November he was persistently aggressive towards both parents. Despite this, they felt he was better and generally happy, spending more time on his own talking imaginatively to himself.

In December 1962 Glyn was placed in the nursery-school class for a trial period but did not fit in. He whimpered continuously and kept repeating the teacher's name to himself. He refused to use the school lavatory and became very anxious and excited whenever he entered or left the classroom. On an educational level, he took no interest in materials provided, save to chew or eat them, and would join in no group activities such as stories or radio programmes. He was, therefore, returned to a therapeutic play group, where he was calm and spent much time on his own playing with plasticine and bricks. His favourite activity was still described as 'provoking an unfavourable response in others'. However, for some time now his toilet habits had been good, and he was felt to be generally less tense and anxious.

The first few months of 1963 brought further slow social improvement. Tense and persistent questioning continued and he was grossly overactive, jumping up and down and flapping his hands while he spoke. He seemed always to be watching for other children's reactions to his behaviour. He constantly needed reassurance about being liked, and swung between periods of cheerfulness and depression. For the first time his talk was concerned with sex and whether certain things were rude. At Easter his home leave followed the familiar pattern of obsessive questioning, aggression, and bed-stripping.

By June Glyn's behaviour seemed to be worsening again. It was impossible to have psychotherapeutic sessions with him, as he became very agitated, jumping up and down flapping his hands and making anxious noises. He was again going to nursery school each morning but did very little, and often had to be returned to the House because of his disruptive behaviour. His July holiday was the most disturbed since admission. He ate everything he picked up: dirt, flowers, grass, and paper. He refused to leave his mother and would not go to bed alone. Most days he would go off alone, take off his trousers and masturbate, producing an erection. If his mother tried to interfere, he would say that he wanted to be rude. Despite all this, he stayed at home for five weeks, and his mother described the holiday as generally happy.

Glyn was now 8 and, in spite of severe psychotic disturbance, was operating with relatively good memory, and very considerable awareness of situations and relationships. After returning from leave he seemed to stabilize over the rest of the year, becoming less tense and more relaxed, and showing less obsessional fearfulness about soiling and wetting. As his school teacher had left, he spent most of this time in a therapeutic play group, where he enjoyed drawing and modelling in plasticine. He was also less aggressive towards the other children and would occasionally play with them or sit quietly watching what was going on.

At Christmas his mother found him more difficult, especially over discipline. She was afraid to take him out, as he would shout and swear at passers-by, and dash out in front of traffic if she let go his hand. On return to West Stowell he slipped back into the old pattern of obsessive, anxious behaviour but was still relaxed. At Easter his parents again found the main difficulty was his embarrassing behaviour in public. On a bus he would suddenly shout 'Why doesn't that man have a haircut?' or 'She's ugly. Will she come home with us?'

In May 1964 new houseparents took over his group. At first Glyn seemed to grow more anxious as a result of this but after a few months would accept affectionate approaches. He still had many toilet obsessions, and would not sit on the lavatory, but rested on his hands. He frequently soiled, usually while in his play group.

By August Glyn had been in the unit for two and a half years. He still showed an overriding fearfulness, especially on certain topics. This was slightly less embracing than formerly, but the apparent improvements over the last year had not changed the basic nature of his condition and behaviour. While on summer holiday his parents noticed that often he was so tense that he could not defecate in the lavatory. He would either go out into the garden or pass a motion in his pants. Treatment continued to aim at reassurance and helping resolve his overriding anxieties and adjust to demands made on him. The diagnosis of childhood psychosis with schizoid features was considered to be confirmed. There was no evidence of a specific organic cause, and his condition seemed likely to be constitutional with a background of vulnerable genetic inheritance and inappropriate early management. His parents seemed to be finding it harder to cope with him and had returned him from his summer holiday after two weeks. At Christmas 1964, however, they found him better, and expressed gratitude for his progress. This followed a calmer period at the unit. During this time he had been tried again in the nursery-school class and fitted in with some difficulties.

For a time at school he showed anxiety, especially over whether the teacher would take him back to the House if he wanted to go. He was very preoccupied with excretory and genital processes, and also with natural phenomena such as the sun, moon, and rain. He constantly provoked aggression from other children, and then appeared to be frightened by it. He liked music and dancing, and showed interest in matching colours and shapes. It was hard to judge his real ability, as he was rarely sufficiently relaxed to reveal it.

After his Christmas holiday Glyn appeared very disturbed, and refused to go back into his family group. When persuaded to, he began to hit himself and then said that his housefather had 'clobbered' him. Within a few weeks, however, he had resettled, and was helping his houseparents with simple jobs. He was still attending the nursery group half-time and was now making good progress. He showed an ambivalent attitude towards his teacher, at times very affectionate and a moment later trying to poke her eyes, although aggression was less marked than in the previous term when he had twice broken her glasses. He now asked for favourite pieces of music, and would sit still for longer periods matching shapes and colours. Towards the middle of the term he once more became very concerned over entering and leaving his classroom, often refusing to do so and standing desperately moaning and flapping if asked to come in. Eventually his teacher tried leading him in, firmly ignoring whatever he said, and he accepted this, apparently grateful for having his mind made up for him. At times he had bouts of anxiety which were so severe as to suggest hallucinatory episodes.

By Easter 1965 it was felt that he was moving forward again, establishing relationships with teacher and houseparents and appearing more relaxed during psychotherapeutic sessions. However, when he went home he regressed. He frequently stripped the bed at night and would remove his trousers and masturbate when there were visitors in the room. His mother reported that she found him impossible to control. On return this behaviour continued. At school he soiled frequently and had to be returned to the House. He was also noticed to be continually fingering his anus. In an attempt to deal directly with this, Glyn was given regular aperients and a record kept of motions passed and frequency of soiling. By the third week he had responded well and seemed happier. By the end of June the soiling had stopped completely. Soon after this he went on leave again.

When he returned to West Stowell he talked as if he had watched his parents having intercourse; he said he had seen his father lie on top of his mother and 'do dirty things'. It seemed unlikely that this was the result of inventive imagination, and possibly reflected once more the extra difficulties that Glyn had to face at home.

In August Glyn had another leave, during which his behaviour was very disturbed. His parents complained of him stripping his bed, tearing sheets and pyjamas, and attacking his mother and the children.

After three and a half years in the unit Glyn's anxiety seemed less often to result in frenzied jumping, but the obsessive questioning persisted unchanged. His themes were basically three: (i) lavatorial and excretory: 'Can I have tea down the toilet?' 'Can I eat shit?'; (ii) sexual/genital: 'Can I be rude?' (in reference to masturbation) 'Will X [housefather or other male staff] prick my wee wee?'; (iii) time and place: 'Where is C group?' 'When will Mr X be on duty?' 'Will I have tea with you?' Later he returned to his older obsession with punishment and being liked.

When upset, Glyn had coughing bouts in which he would double up and stick his fingers into his anus. These often lasted for two or three minutes and during them he would be so absorbed that he would not respond to any words addressed to him. At times he was very contented and wore a peaceful smile on his face, usually at bed-time in his family group and when listening to music in school. At other times he would produce long complex comments and remarks over a wide range of topics in response to conversation.

Towards the end of the year Glyn suffered a number of blows. His mother went into hospital for a hysterectomy and soon after this his teacher went into hospital for an operation. Meanwhile the senior nursing staff, a married couple who had been in charge of the unit for the past five years and two houseparents left, so that Glyn's housemother had to supervise another group. A few weeks later his houseparents left and his group for a time had no permanent intensive care staff. Glyn was manifestly affected by these disruptions and began to soil himself regularly, to regurgitate food, and smear faeces. On a number of occasions he stripped his bed and tore the sheets or threw them out of the window.

At Christmas he had the most disturbed leave since admission. He was obsessionally anxious over going to the toilet and wet his bed every night, as well as often soiling and smearing. He was also aggressive towards his mother, who was convalescent, and she wrote saying he had been absolutely impossible.

On return in January 1966 he was very agitated. At school, where a temporary teacher was in charge, he soiled two or three times a week, frequently smearing his faeces. In an attempt to ease this he was allowed to indulge in water play and to paint himself, both of which activities he appeared to enjoy greatly. However, he was still obsessed with excretion and would strain his abdomen putting his fingers into his anus. He took no interest in toilet cleanliness and did not participate in cleaning himself. Towards the end of February he started tearing his clothes again and had to be put into strong garments, as he destroyed any other he wore.

Easter leave was even worse than Christmas. He showed no self-control and was constantly ripping clothes and sheets until he had destroyed all his mother had put on his bed. He had also started to eat his faeces, which he said other children at West Stowell did. His mother wrote a frenzied note saying she could not bear to have him home again. Later, however, after visiting Glyn and spending an afternoon with him she changed her mind. On return from this leave he was very restless, tearing his clothes, smearing and eating his faeces, and throwing bedding out of his dormitory window. For a short period he would speak only in a whisper, and at one stage appeared to have lost all speech, making no response to any approach. He was very depressed and at times appeared hallucinated. He came out of this phase quite suddenly, and showed no signs of regression afterwards. He was now smearing less but continued to tear clothes to shreds, including specially reinforced shirts. He appeared to like a pair of long trousers and left these alone. In May he recommenced school, where his teacher found him to be in much the same state as when she first had him, two years earlier, though his anxieties now seemed rather more concentrated. He was a disruptive influence and brought much of the normal work of the class to a halt. In his family group he also easily upset others, and led one or two children to copy him, possibly in order to get the attention his behaviour inevitably brought. However disturbed he was, Glyn always seemed to be aware of the effect his actions were having, and to aim deliberately at creating hostility towards himself.

By May 1966 Glyn was 10½ and remained a very disturbed child, although recovering from the excessive behaviour of the previous few months. He had been withdrawn from the nursery-school group and now spent his time in a play group. For a short period he was kept in bed during mornings in an attempt to diminish stimulation, and given tranquillizers by day, and sedatives at night. The tearing had almost stopped, but he was showing bouts of aggression, especially towards female staff. In one such episode he injured the shoulder of one of the temporary staff. Questioning now circled around hurting people, and sleeping in the paddling pool. At the end of a month medication was changed, with better response. Glyn was more relaxed, ready to play, and less aggressive. However, it was uncertain how long this improvement would last. Despite changes in his pattern of behaviour and periods of calm lucid conversation and cheerful play, there was no indication of any real progress and long-term prognosis was poor.

9. GUY

Born 1 December 1953

Admitted: 7 August 1962

Reason for admission: referred from the children's unit of a long-stay psychiatric hospital as a psychotic child in need of intensive treatment

Height: 4 ft 4 in   Weight: 4 st 6 lb

IQ: 58 and 70 (Terman-Merrill, 1962)

EEG: normal

Skull X-ray: some bridging of cells; otherwise within normal limits

Bone-age: *c*. 10 years when 9

Treatment: Child-centred intensive care in family group

　August 1962–February 1966: regressed nurtural care in therapeutic play group

　March 1966 onwards: nursery class

Guy was referred by a consultant after a year's observation as a possibly deaf, withdrawn child. Investigations suggested he was neither deaf nor subnormal, but psychotic and in need of intensive environmental treatment. No organic basis for his condition had

154

been revealed. His mother had totally rejected him and he was under the guardianship of an aunt.

Guy was a planned and wanted child, and his mother had a normal pregnancy. Birth was three weeks overdue, and he weighed 9 lb, but there were no complications. He was breast-fed for three months, and then changed to a bottle with no trouble. He smiled at 4 weeks, sat up at 9 months and crawled at 11 months. A photograph at 10 months shows an attractive, healthy, and apparently normal child. He is said to have been a lazy and placid baby but there is no definite indication that he was abnormally passive.

After the first year his progress was slower. He is said to have fallen from a window onto a concrete path at 15 months old, but there is no evidence that he was seriously injured. He did not walk until 2 years and responded to toilet-training only after the age of 3.

Until he was $3\frac{1}{2}$ Guy lived with his parents. He was mostly looked after by a 15-year-old domestic who had many other duties, and could not spend much time with him. At about 18 months he was unable to speak, and moved around on two feet and one hand. It was also noticed that he rarely played with toys, although he took an old blanket and a battered teddy bear to bed with him. He was always an active child and as he grew older he became restless and overactive. At other times he would sit alone in silent self-absorption.

When he was $3\frac{1}{2}$ the parents emigrated, taking their children with them. From this time his mother's attitude began to change from indifference to open rejection and hostility.

Guy's mother was mentally disturbed. Emotionally overactive, with wide mood swings, she acted out her feelings. She said she disliked bringing up children and longed for a free life.

Soon after emigrating Guy started to attend occasionally a special unit for retarded children, but nothing is known of his progress there. He had still not developed speech, and his parents sought help. Opinions varied. One doctor said that he was normal apart from his speech defect; another thought he was partially deaf and fitted a hearing aid. However, his parents knew he could not be deaf, as he readily imitated tunes heard from the radio. Later tests confirmed that he had no significant hearing loss. His mother, rejecting of his disabilities, considered him strong-willed and disobedient, and often punished him as such. When she hit him he reacted by attacking his sister, or anyone else nearby.

155

In the spring of 1959 Guy went to a children's health centre for investigation of his abnormal behaviour and lack of speech. Physical examination revealed no organic defect; skull X-ray and EEG were both normal. Hearing was tested, and no impairment was found. It was noted that he liked to hum and that he sang tunefully in a modulated voice. The specialist who examined him commented on his limited comprehension of the spoken word, and said that he showed 'a marked difficulty in sound perception and organization of sound perception to produce adequate responses'.

After consultation with the child-guidance clinic which referred him, he was diagnosed as mentally retarded with a primary inability to organize perceptual stimuli so as to make a vocal response to situations; not as a juvenile schizophrenic or autistic. The suggestion was that he had an abnormality of the central nervous system, of unknown origin. Residential care was recommended.

Meanwhile Guy was visited by his aunt, who was distressed at his backwardness and his mother's rejecting attitude. She, therefore, took him back to England. She was ready to include him in her family, and wanted first to have him assessed medically, as she was distrustful of the hospital reports.

In December 1959 Guy was admitted to hospital. Skull X-ray and EEG again proved normal, and a urine test showed no indication of phenylketonuria. He was described as 'a deprived child, but one who displayed signs of psychotic behaviour'.

On the hospital's recommendation he was admitted to a children's home where he was seen regularly by the consultant who referred him there. His aunt visited him frequently. He stayed there from January 1960 until September 1961, when he was transferred to another hospital. While there he was investigated in the deaf unit, and normal hearing found. Various intelligence tests were administered and, though he showed little interest in the tests, he was given an intelligence rating as high as 70 on the Merrill-Palmer Scale non-verbal items, and it was suggested that he might prove educable at a school for the educationally subnormal. During these years his aunt had him home for short leaves, most of which were very stormy. He screamed much of the time, threw food, and tore curtains and sheets. The worst occasion was in March 1961, when his father visited England and took Guy to stay with his grandparents. After one and a half days of continual screaming and running away, he had to take him back to his aunt's where he was calmer. On return to the children's home he was said to have been desperate, screaming, and constantly wetting and soiling himself. After this his father refused to consider taking him home and felt that he should not visit at all.

Guy was admitted to West Stowell on 7 August 1962 at the age of $8\frac{1}{2}$, a large blond boy, still unable to speak but expressing himself with high-pitched screams when upset. His toilet habits were reasonably good, he could dress and undress himself, and was able to eat tidily with a knife and fork. On admission he was very disturbed and seemed upset at the change of environment. During physical examination he was highly nervous and unco-operative and panicked very readily when any unfamiliar move was made to examine him.

In the first few weeks Guy showed little sign of settling. He rejected overtures from staff and refused to play. If the atmosphere of his play group was disturbed, he responded by sudden outbursts of screaming, or by aggressiveness towards a younger child. He showed a number of odd mannerisms, rolling his eyes, rotating his body while balanced on one leg, plucking at his pullover and manipulating the biceps of female members of staff (the only spontaneous contact he made with adults). He was placed in a family group where his houseparents gave him a great deal of direct personal contact and provided a calm structured atmosphere. Primarily treatment was to consist chiefly of regressed nurtural care in a therapeutic play group, where he might be able to form a basic relationship on an infantile level.

After a month or so, during which his toilet habits and self-care regressed, Guy stabilized, but by the end of the year had shown no indication of moving forward. Relations with adults were of a semi-mechanical nature, though he enjoyed vigorous play. He accepted the other children but was jealous of their relations with adults. His behaviour varied from overactivity and excitement to periods of self-absorbed passivity. There were sudden outbursts of agitation and screaming which seemed to reflect real anxiety; at other times he sat quietly showing a morbid interest in his own body, plucking at this clothes or picking his mouth until it bled. His expression was at once blank and perturbed, and the blankness seemed to be a cover for a very disturbed inner state of mind rather than a simple lack of mental processes.

At the beginning of 1963 he was transferred to the play group

M

which contained the less outgoing children, as it had been noted that he was made uneasy by noise and movement. He seemed happier after this, and could be persuaded to spend some time on cutting paper into strips and other constructive play. He was still uneasy regarding the other children and shrank back at the approach of even a small quiet child. He was very apprehensive of the consulting-room, and was usually unhappy to leave his play group. It was remarked that only in the context of a room he knew, and in the presence of people with whom he was very familiar, did Guy show any sign of relaxation. There were signs of him reaching this stage with his houseparents and play therapist, but even with them a disturbance in routine or concern with another child could send him off into a bout of overactivity and screaming.

By May he seemed to be making occasional contact. He would smile in response to approaches by staff, and make affectionate contact with some. If frustrated or upset, he reacted with a high-pitched scream. He had by now recovered from a further period of regression in toilet and dressing habits. In August he had a disastrous leave. In addition to the usual difficulties and wet beds, he urinated over the breakfast table and his bed, on both occasions with apparently deliberate provocation as he had waited until his aunt entered the room before starting. Later in the year his aunt became ill, and wrote saying she would be unable to have him home any more.

At West Stowell Guy showed little change in attitude. He usually appeared disinterested and showed little response to affection, beyond turning his head when his name was called, and offering his cheek when asked for a kiss. In his play group he still resisted any activity apart from paper-cutting, and preferred to sit alone, picking fluffy wool off his clothes or a blanket, or playing with great absorption with his spittle, which he would flick between his thumb and fore-finger. He enjoyed going for walks, and readily joined in the PT sessions, despite the noise and movement. However, when he was 10, in December 1963, he could be said only to have made slight forward movement, and remained exceptionally retarded for his age.

Guy spent Christmas at the children's home where he had lived for eighteen months after first coming to England. On return to West Stowell he continued for some months with little change in his behaviour. Staff had changed, and he seemed lost and unable to do anything constructive without the close support he had had before.

In May 1964 new houseparents took over his family group. They found Guy in a very disturbed state, frequently screaming, incontinent of urine, sick after most meals. He rejected offers of affection and seemed unwilling to communicate. After a few months he had become sufficiently used to them to enjoy rough play and chases. He also accepted minor physical approaches, such as hair-combing or being helped with a jigsaw puzzle. In the autumn pony-riding was introduced as a regular event for the children. He showed great interest in this, and obviously found the experience a pleasant one, though he would become very disturbed before his turn. Another experience which aroused interest in him was watching films taken of the children at play in the garden. This seemed to suggest that the use of heightened experience might be of importance in treating him. His early years had been marked by a complete lack of normal affection, and much of his life since then had been spent in institutions.

In August he spent two weeks at a holiday home and three days with his aunt, who found him highly disturbed. She reported that he had screamed frequently without cause but had played less with his spittle. After his leave he was still disturbed, jumping up and down in an agitated fashion if anyone unfamiliar approached him to take him to the toilet, or guide him to the meal table. In bed he hid under the bed-clothes. Often he behaved as if he were in a delusional state, and ordinary approaches were misinterpreted as potentially aggressive acts.

Towards the end of the year his behaviour calmed down again and he showed some signs of developing his initially good contact with his new houseparents. In the family group he helped with push-ing the food trolley. His clothes-picking had stopped and his patho-logical preoccupation with plucking at the area around his mouth also ceased. His new mannerism was to move around on one foot with a hopping motion. Toilet habits remained variable, but he was usually dry and clean with routine supervision and raising at night.

In January 1965 Guy's father wrote, in response to a letter from his aunt, saying that there were no suitable placements for Guy abroad near his family and implying that he did not really want to make arrangements for him. Guy's mother, he said, would have nothing to do with him, and would not have him at home, while the only available hospital had a long waiting list and was very under-staffed as well. He was told that Guy would have to leave West

159

Stowell eventually and that, therefore, it was important for him to keep contact with relatives. Guy had made a little further progress at West Stowell and needed the personal interest of at least one person over a long period. It was considered that he should be able eventually to live in the community as a handicapped person, and should have a long-term contact in preparation for this. His father finally agreed to have Guy's name put down for a special residential school.

At Easter Guy went for a week to his holiday home, and later spent a few days in London with his houseparents. During this time they found him no trouble, and said he was much better than he had been at West Stowell. He had wet his bed once only, and had had no screaming attacks, although staying in a strange house. They had been able to take him to the cinema and on bus rides, all of which he enjoyed. He had coped well with meals, excusing himself to go to the toilet, and even helping to wash up after meals. Towards the end of the holiday he seemed to be making a far greater use of speech sounds in an attempt to communicate.

The promise of these few days was not fulfilled after his return to West Stowell, but he did seem slowly to be becoming a more competent and interested person. His aunt found him less agitated when he stayed with her for a few days in August, but he still had not really emerged from his passive state and there was no speech. Hopes that he might return home were lessened by an excited letter from his mother saying she could never bear to see him again.

Guy seemed now to be making slow progress and it was expected that he would be able to join the nursery class soon. In the autumn he responded well to a party that was held in the unit although he had been very disturbed beforehand during the preparations. He ate well at the table with his family group and later joined in dancing with his houseparents. A similar reaction at a later Christmas party confirmed the impression that such experiences were of importance to him. Towards the end of the year his houseparents left. The housefather, a trained mental nurse, had taken a special interest in him, and Guy missed him. He had a disturbed holiday and on return after Christmas was found to have picked away much of the skin around his mouth.

In the first few weeks after return Guy was easily upset by noises and had to be taken out of his therapeutic play group. New houseparents came in April, and it was hoped that he might eventually build up a good relationship with them. His first reaction was to be upset by any change in routine. Once at breakfast, when he was served with shredded wheat instead of the usual cornflakes, he became agitated and tipped over the table, which upset other members of the group. His housemother, who was alone in charge, went to comfort another child, at which Guy butted her in the back with his head. Ten minutes later he was quietly sitting and eating his breakfast.

In May 1966 Guy, now 12½, was still suffering from a severe psychotic condition. No speech had developed, though he would copy the sound stresses of his name. If left to play alone in familiar surroundings, he was content for long periods. He would become absorbed in water play, in flicking pieces of fluff from his pullover, or throwing grass onto the road outside the unit, often laughing happily to himself while doing so. Yet at other times he would suddenly become agitated, screaming and running away as if hallucinated, and rejecting approaches from even familiar staff. Once, when a large party was visiting the unit, he became so disturbed that he stripped off all his clothing and upset tables in the schoolroom. At school he was now settling well and responding to personal attention from his teacher, enjoying jigsaws and showing some skill in matching shapes. However, his general level of operation was still very retarded and there seemed little prospect of him living outside hospital for some years, especially in the absence of individual interest in him.

10. JOSEPH

Born: 30 January 1955
Admitted: 2 September 1963
Discharged: 23 November 1964
Reason for admission: aggressive behaviour and emotional immaturity; excluded from school and proving very difficult at children's home
Height: 4 ft 7½ in   Weight: 5 st 4 lb
IQ: 100 (1961)
EEG: not taken

Skull X-ray: normal
Bone-age: 8 years when 8
Treatment: child-centred intensive care in family group
  formal school class

Joseph was referred to West Stowell from a child-guidance clinic, as a major behaviour problem at the children's home where he had been living for the previous eight months. He was recommended for a short period of intensive residential treatment, having been excluded from primary school because of his conduct, which included ramming children with desks, and stealing their bicycles.

Joseph was the illegitimate child of an Anglo-Indian manual labourer and a subnormal girl. His mother was living in a Home at the time of his birth and had a number of hysterical fits during early pregnancy. She received phenobarbitone, and had an uncomplicated pregnancy apart from this until the last month when she developed toxaemia. Labour was surgically induced, but delivery was normal. Birth weight was 6 lb 13 oz.

Joseph lived with his mother for just over a month, after which he was received into local-authority care and placed in a residential nursery. His mother did not visit, and her family refused to let her bring Joseph home. However, his father's mother took an interest in him, visited him regularly, and offered to have him with her. In March 1955, when he was 14 months old, he was boarded out with her by the children's department.

Joseph's grandmother was an Anglo-Indian of noticeably fragile build. She gave birth to his father when she was only 14 years old, and had had two other children, both daughters. She came to England to join her 'husband', only to find that he was already married. At the time she offered to have Joseph she was living on National Assistance. One of her daughters was living at home with an illegitimate child, while the other was married but constantly talked of leaving her husband.

Joseph subsequently saw nothing of his mother and only rarely his father, who had married and started a family. He totally rejected his son, but Joseph later seemed very proud of his father, often boasting about his anti-social behaviour.

Joseph's early milestones seem to have been normal, but by the time he was 3 he was showing aggression towards children in the

162

neighbourhood. His grandmother tried to stop him from playing with other children, because she said they bullied him, but this seems to have been the reverse of the truth. She seems to have been the one person with whom Joseph developed any sort of relationship in his early years.

In 1960 Joseph started school. He would not accept classroom discipline, made no attempt to learn anything, and was frequently aggressive towards other children in his class. Towards the end of the year he was referred to a child-guidance clinic. He was unable to count, could read no more than two or three words, and would only copy his name, but his intelligence quotient, on test in 1961, rated as 100.

Joseph seemed to live in a world of aggressive fantasy, reflected in his drawing, which was vividly colourful and violent. His dreams were full of action and excitement: houses on fire, horses running away, men being killed. At the clinic he was summed up as a very disturbed child venting his disturbance on other children at school by taking their belongings and trying to hurt them.

After two years he was excluded from school. Behaviour had steadily worsened and he had been seen to attack children, hitting them with skipping rope handles and pushing desks at them. He had also taken several bicycles. He was placed in a children's home from which, as a Catholic, he attended a Catholic day school. He made no progress, and behaved in a similar manner to that which had led to his exclusion from school previously. At the children's home he was aggressive, smashed toys belonging to other children, and made no relationships. In June 1963 he was again seen at the child-guidance clinic and considered in need of residential intensive psychiatric treatment.

Joseph was brought for interview to West Stowell by his grandmother, whom he called 'mother', and a children's home houseparent. He appeared to have great inner tension, which he expressed by hostility towards child rivals and controlling adults. Considerable discrepancy existed between his infantile emotional state and physical and mental abilities. Prognosis seemed unfavourable unless he received intensive psychotherapeutic management, and he was accordingly admitted to West Stowell House in September 1963 as a short-stay patient.

On admission Joseph was 8½, a tall well-built Eurasian, with dark

163

brown hair and eyes. Personal habits were all good, but he was very retarded educationally. He could count up to ten and recognize a few words, but little more. He was self-assertive, with a positive manner, and rejected control. He settled into West Stowell with an air of detached independence. At night he tended to play up and take a long time to settle, disturbing the other children in his bedroom. He was placed in the formal school class, as it was clearly important to make some progress with his education, so that he could fit into a school on leaving West Stowell. Apart from this, treatment was to consist of intensive management based on acceptance and tolerance of Joseph as a person, and refusal to respond with aggression to his aggressive acts towards staff or children.

Soon after his arrival there was a series of staff changes and this may have been a factor in his initially disturbed behaviour. Joseph made good contact with an older boy who was admitted to the unit soon after he was, also for a conduct disorder, and tended to be led by him. At school they proved difficult to control, and Joseph, especially, made no response to teaching. As a result of this he was moved to a therapeutic play group, as he was distracting other children from their work. Here the regressed nurtural care approach was tried so that he could work through some basic personal relationships. His other need was for the intimate life of a family group, but his houseparents left soon after his admission, and new ones had not yet come. During his stay in the play group his behaviour continued to be as contrary as it had been in school. He would ask to go to the toilet and then run off. In fact he did not receive regressed nurtural care, because staff found he resented any approaches of this sort. However, in the play group, he was receiving child-centred care, and at times there were signs that he was affected by the interest shown in him.

One of Joseph's basic difficulties was that formerly he had been either resented or disliked by most adults, because of his egotistical outgoing behaviour. It was, therefore, encouraging to find that some staff members found him a rewarding child. In these first few months Joseph's attitude was guarded and suspicious, but his behaviour was rarely as difficult as reports from previous placings had suggested. His various escapades seemed to reflect boredom as much as hostility to authority.

In December 1963 his grandmother and Child Care Officer paid a first visit. He responded well to this and seemed to enjoy their coming. He spent Christmas in his previous children's home, where he was considered much improved and had expressed his happiness at West Stowell. He was obviously looking forward to going back to West Stowell, and told the staff it was because he was allowed to do what he liked there. He spent Christmas and Boxing Day with his grandmother, who also noted an improvement in his behaviour and said that everyone had had a very happy holiday as a result of this.

After Christmas Joseph's behaviour worsened, especially in regard to his attitude towards other children. Asked why he attacked them, he showed no remorse and said it was because they annoyed him, or were nasty and hit other children themselves. His behaviour so deteriorated during this period that a member of staff described him as 'unlikable and unliked both by children and adults'. Many of his actions seemed provocative: he would watch until an adult's back was turned and then attack a small child, afterwards denying it. At other times he would be deliberately damaging, by turning on taps and flooding a room or breaking crockery, often apparently in order to get attention. Staff were encouraged to accept his wilful behaviour as indicative of a need for a relationship and so help break down his resentment against adults.

In the spring new houseparents came, affording an opportunity to use a parenting approach to Joseph. They found him hostile at first and constantly trying to provoke them to anger. He dominated and controlled the family group, disrupting it with ease. The houseparents, therefore, made special efforts to get him to play a part in running the group with them, and found that he enjoyed this. It also helped the other children to emerge as individuals. After some months he was still a dominant figure in the group but used his position to help the younger and less able members.

He was now back in the school class, where he had announced on his first day that he was a naughty boy, and then proceeded to demonstrate the fact. This time his teacher persevered with him, despite the disrupting effect on the other children, and gradually he began to accept the classroom situation. He was still unstable and aggressive when frustrated.

There was evidence that Joseph's conduct disorder was a complex one. He was sensitive about his colour, and this seemed to be one element in his aggressiveness. On one occasion another child was taunting him, and finally vomited over him. Joseph went wild at this and punched him about, pushing him on the floor and kicking him. At this stage a visitor to the House, who was watching, called him a 'black bastard'. This upset Joseph even more, and he needed much reassurance from his houseparents, who were treating his aggression as symptomatic of real needs. He later confided to his housefather that the children at the children's home had called him 'Golliwog' and his concern was revealed by the ambivalent attitude he showed to a toy golliwog he possessed, which he cherished, but would also treat violently and had once 'hanged'.

In the summer Joseph went to the children's home again. Staff said he was still aggressive but less so than before. At West Stowell he was behaving much more maturely, especially in the family group. At school, too, he showed more interest in learning, though if he did any work, or behaved well for a period, he felt bound to make up for this by a bout of rowdiness. He liked reading, and showed an interest in history and geography, as well as an aptitude for mechanical things. He now provided few management problems, and could be trusted to carry out work on his own.

Joseph was now near the point of being ready to leave West Stowell. His outlook was normal and there were no neurotic or psychotic traits in his behaviour. A place was obtained at a school for maladjusted children. It was intended that he should be introduced to his new school gradually by means of a series of visits, culminating in a final transfer after Christmas. However, the headmaster insisted that he should be transferred immediately or not at all, so that Joseph was moved rather suddenly at the end of November, missing the nativity play for which he had been rehearsing and Christmas festivities at West Stowell, to which he had been looking forward. There was no alternative to discharging him, though the situation seemed one of 'moral blackmail'. The problem over his discharge was further aggravated by the headmaster's refusal to allow the Child Care Officer, whom Joseph knew well, to visit him in the first month.

Not surprisingly, Joseph proved a considerable problem at his new placing. Punishment at the school consisted of being made to stand in the hall, or being given a plain supper, and he was punished several times. He showed no overt resentment at this treatment, and at times appeared to go out of his way to invite it.

166

After one term and a few weeks he was excluded, as not being manageable, and returned to live with his grandmother for a trial period. The children's home was available if this failed. On being visited, he was found to be cheerful and self-contained, denying the behaviour which had led to his exclusion from school. However, he seemed to have lost the contact with adults which had emerged in the latter part of his stay at West Stowell. He now needed more structured control than West Stowell could offer, but it was important this should be combined with a recognition of his emotional needs.

On follow-up, in May 1966, Joseph, who was now 11 years old, was at a Catholic residential school for the educationally subnormal, where he had taken his mother's name. Contact had been renewed with his mother who visited him occasionally. The headmaster of the school reported that his work and conduct were satisfactory and that he was making fairly good progress all round. He was a keen and useful footballer and had also joined the school Army Cadet force. He was enjoying his spare time and had a number of friends. It seemed that he had found a suitable placing and was fulfilling the promise he showed on leaving West Stowell House. Contact was being maintained with his father's family and supporting social agencies, he was spending holidays with his grandmother, and prognosis was relatively satisfactory.

11. NEVILLE

Born: 12 December 1953
Admitted: 8 November 1960
Readmitted: February 1961
Reason for admission: overactive, manneristic behaviour; unmanageable at home, difficult at school. Father receiving ECT treatment for depression
Height: 3 ft 9½ in   Weight: 3 st
IQ: 79 (1960)
EEG: not taken
Skull X-ray: within normal limits
Bone-age: *c.* 8 years when 8

Treatment: Child-centred intensive care in family group
  November 1960–April 1961: regressed nurtural care
  May 1961–September 1963: nursery class
  September 1963–October 1964: regressed nurtural care
  October 1964–April 1966: formal school class
  April 1966 onwards: village C.P. School

When Neville was first seen by the writer at 6½ he was making only slow progress at a local private school and was often quite unmanageable at home. His parents were reluctant to lose him but eventually agreed to temporary admission to West Stowell in November 1960. Two weeks later they took him home, but in the following February asked for readmission on a long-term basis.

When six months' pregnant Neville's mother had a haemorrhage, and a month before her confinement contracted pleurisy. Birth was three weeks premature but was fairly easy. Neville weighed 6 lb 4 oz and was 'poor, limp and grey'. He was treated in an oxygen tent and his mother did not see him for the first few days.

She partly breast-fed him for six weeks but then relied entirely on the bottle. He was resistant to toilet-training for a long time and refused to defecate in the lavatory, although quite happy to urinate there. He had sat up at 10 months, and walked at 16 months, but was very timid about this and asked for support long after he needed it. Speech was very late, articulation poor, and he did not use words properly until he was 4. He did not feed himself until aged 2½, having to be bribed with sweets to do so, but later fed well.

His mother said that he had never been a 'cuddly child', but did not feel that he was in any way abnormal until he was 2 or 3. She recalled that at 18 months he had been left at his grandmother's for a few hours during which he had cried all the time, but that he had usually been all right if left.

From the age of 3 onwards Neville showed strong powers of observation. When he could talk he would refer to changes in curtains and furniture in relatives' houses, and even before this seemed very aware of changes in the position of things. He was frightened whenever the family went to a strange place, and would become very excited and overactive. This persisted until he went to school. By the time he was 5 his speech was developing but often seemed rather odd. He would walk about saying 'Neville's dying; Neville's very ill'. He was very fond of water play, and his parents seemed to have allowed him to throw water about freely, even if it entailed flooding the kitchen.

Neville's parents delayed sending him back to school, as they felt he might be rather difficult. He eventually started at a local private school, when he was $5\frac{3}{4}$. He had been given some teaching at home, and could recognize letters although he usually refused to concentrate. At school he was very restless, and the teachers found it hard to get him to co-operate in anything. After two terms he could do simple sums and was on the first reader. He would copy words from the board and then scribble them out. Often, for no reason, he would get excited and knock over his desk or sweep another child's books on to the floor. At times this behaviour reached the point of disrupting the class, and there was talk of excluding him. In April 1960, at the headmistress's suggestion, he was seen by the writer for assessment of his mental state.

Neville was now $6\frac{1}{2}$, and small for his age. He was overactive but seemed less disturbed than most children at West Stowell House. Admission was agreed if parents and teachers felt he was too much for them, but his parents felt that he might regress in the company of more disturbed children. Out-patient care was provided initially, therefore, to obtain a clearer picture of his condition. Over the next few months the likelihood of an organic factor in Neville's excitability emerged. His overactivity and contrariness seemed to be of an impulsive nature, and he seemed to have an unusually irregular skull. Periods of restlessness were followed by days in which he would sit still and be able to draw correct plans of his father's farm.

During the summer term Neville made relatively good progress at school and seemed stabler all round, but when he returned after the summer holiday to a new classroom and teacher he was upset and became very excited and interfered with the other children's work. He developed a cold, and his parents used this as an excuse to keep him at home for a time. He now refused to dress and undress himself or to use the lavatory and demanded constant attention, which he received. On returning to school he had regressed to his previous state, and in November his parents agreed to temporary admission to West Stowell. Behaviour at home had continued to be unpredictable and often provocative; throwing ink on the carpet, putting books on the fire, or flooding the kitchen. He showed no response to punishment or commands. His mother had recently had a baby, and his father had been receiving treatment for depression, so neither was really capable of coping well with Neville.

When seen again prior to admission both his parents were concerned to stress that he was not mentally defective, though there might be some 'pressure on the brain'. His father had recovered from his depression but still seemed anxious and at a loss. Neville's latest school report had been slightly better, and they were inclined to keep him at home and pretend he was getting better, but finally agreed that he needed investigation and consented to admission for a fortnight.

Neville then entered West Stowell in November 1960; he was to stay for up to three weeks and to go home every weekend. On admission he was very unhappy and cried more than usual. He would not mix with the other children and spent much of his time on his own, walking about stiffly with his hands behind his back, talking to himself. He was placed in the school class, as the play group was rather too boisterous for him. Speech was very poorly articulated, although content and use were normal. There was an occasional tendency towards echolalia. While at West Stowell Neville had transient glycosuria and was investigated for possible abnormal carbohydrate metabolism, but all tests proved negative. At the end of a fortnight the picture that emerged was of a child of average intelligence, congenitally retarded in personality development, and handicapped in educational achievement by temperamental instability which led to poor concentration, overactivity, and excitability. He seemed also to be suffering from being too closely attached to an anxious and over-solicitous mother. He did not show the abnormal behaviour reported elsewhere.

Neville returned home at the end of November, and arrangements for regular out-patient care were made. His parents were advised to keep in contact and consider the possibility of a longer stay if there were signs of worsening in his behaviour pattern. At Christmas he was manageable over the actual festivities but then became very disturbed, pushing over cups at the table, spluttering food from his mouth, tearing up books, emptying drawers, and throwing toys at his younger brother. His behaviour, while never overtly aggressive, was constantly provocative. On returning to school his teachers felt that he was making no progress and had even lost some of the skills he had developed. In mental arithmetic, previously one of his better subjects, he now used his quickness deliberately to think up a wrong answer and so draw attention to himself. If this did not work, he would throw his books on the floor or urinate over another child.

His father now decided that Neville might after all benefit from residential treatment and he was readmitted to West Stowell. He seemed more agitated than previously and the psychotic elements in his conduct were more apparent. His toilet and eating habits were good, and, apart from restless, frequently silly giggling behaviour, he presented few management problems, especially in comparison with other children in the unit. He was placed in a therapeutic play group where a period of regressed nurtural care would help him following the break from his parents. His parents were encouraged to visit but not to take him home for a month. Neville talked a lot about 'going home', but this was considered unduly disturbing to both child and parents initially. In his play groups he would not mix with other children but sat quietly on his own doing jigsaw puzzles.

At no time during the first three months in West Stowell was he as disturbed as at home. He went home most weekends, and his week circled round this, anticipating and recalling with obsessive interest the exact time he was going to be, or had been, collected. At times he became noticeably tense over small incidents, and on such occasions his arm and leg muscles would stiffen and he would regress to an infantile giggling level. Generally, however, he seemed less anxious and in the play group spent much of his time doing sums and undertaking other activities beyond the level of most children in his group. It was, therefore, decided to transfer him to the nursery-school class after Easter.

Easter leave was uneventful and it was now arranged that he should go home every fortnight, his parents visiting in between. He did not settle at school as well as had been expected and showed as much provocative behaviour as at his former school: knocking over desks, turning on taps, and transiently exposing himself. He would play dominoes, but refused to match letters or do sums, although it was known he could do them. If given paper to work on, he frequently tore it up. This continued over the year and it was felt that in some ways his behaviour worsened as he became more accustomed to the unit. In psychotherapeutic sessions he avoided direct conversation and talked obsessively about how many minutes were left before he would have to go. In such sessions his behaviour was frequently impulsive and provocative: he would throw sand in the writer's face, urinate on the floor, or smash a toy, usually asking whether he was allowed to do this. In the House he continually watched other children but refused to join their games. In August he had been placed in a family group and seemed to be benefiting from this. After a month or so he began to talk spontaneously to his house-parents, often about time matters, but more frequently of his family, apart from his brother, of whom he seemed very jealous. Ritual ques-tions expressing anxieties and tensions, were received sympathetically and given appropriate answers. By the end of the year they found that he had gained sufficient self-confidence to be 'cheeky' to them.

Just before he was due to go home for Christmas he went through a period of rolling about on the floor kicking and shrieking until his mother arrived to take him home. His leave was not unduly dis-turbed, although he pulled wallpaper off the walls of his bedroom.

Neville was now 8 and still small for his age. He was overactive, at times almost hypomanic, but seemed generally cheerful and affec-tionate. Over the next few months his behaviour changed little, apart from a slow maturation in the context of his family group, where he showed less impulsive and provocative behaviour. At Easter his parents noted a great interest in books. He also spent long periods with an illustrated children's dictionary, studying the pic-tures and reading the captions.

Soon after this Neville's family group broke up and this had an unsettling effect on him. His behaviour was still conformative much of the time, but the eruptive periods occurred more frequently. Alongside this, he appeared to be becoming more aware of his own behaviour. He would say that he felt the giggling coming on, and explain away a provocative act by saying that another child had made him be silly. He still failed to make any progress at school, and seemed unable even to reach the standard described at the private school attended before admission. His weekends at home had been proving a strain on his parents and had a disturbing effect on him, so it was decided that he should go home for brief trips on Saturday and Sunday, but not stay overnight. As his parents lived near, this arrangement was practicable. His latest interest was in maps and the passage of the sun in the sky. He was able to tell the sun's position at any time of day and recite times of sunset and sunrise for long periods ahead. When taken out in the car by his father he liked to act as guide, and showed a remarkable ability at reading road signs and following maps.

By the beginning of 1963 Neville had spent two years in the unit. His parents thought he was better controlled, but little real change had been noticed at West Stowell, beyond a growing familiarity with the place, and a little less impulsiveness associated with some physical and emotional maturation. He still became very disturbed during therapeutic sessions, which sometimes had to be terminated early because he got so excited. Sometimes he would say under his breath 'I must be good', but a moment later would be throwing sand around or urinating on the floor. At home he became upset at any accident, such as a broken cup; once after a cup had been broken at a neighbour's he ran home impetuously and smashed a window.

His houseparents felt he was slowly making progress. He was less easily upset and did not appear so obsessed with toilet matters. In September his school teacher left, and he was temporarily placed in a therapeutic play group. Reaction was satisfactory and it was decided that he might benefit from being kept in such a group for a period, as he had failed to respond to the classroom situation.

Neville was now 10 and had spent a fortnight at home over Christmas during which his main interest had been in the radio and following the times of programmes in the *Radio Times*. His manneristic behaviour, whenever he was visited, continued. His latest trait was the use of obscenities. When excited he jumped up and down shouting 'shit' in a shrill, unconvincing voice, and even in his play group he often used letters to spell out a swear word. At times he was able to behave in a calm and normal way; a girl patient went to tea with her mother at Neville's home, and he behaved well throughout. His map interest was maintained, and he continued to give the impression of being a basically intelligent child even though his psychotic conduct disorder continued at a severe level.

Although in many ways Neville appeared too able for a therapeutic play group, he did, in fact, show more signs of using his ability in this context than he had at school. He could place any county on a blank map of Britain and was able to write a few words if given encouragement. He still refused all contact with other children, preferring to walk around with arms held behind his back and eyes looking at the floor, if he were not specifically occupied. His parents visited regularly and towards the end of 1964 offered to take a number of children to tea at their farm. The tea itself was a great success, with everyone apparently enjoying themselves very much. On the way back Neville got very excited and threw both sandals and his father's pocket watch out of the car window.

Now almost 11, Neville's attitude and behaviour seemed largely to depend on the situation in which he found himself. He tended to be agitated at home, while in his family group he was relatively quiet and stable, although he still would not mix with other children and showed only occasional approaches to his houseparents. As soon as he was upset or excited his behaviour reverted to the familiar pattern of asking for drinks and visits to the toilet, which often ended in shrieked obscenities. The psychotic process had been worsened but he was in fairly good contact with his environment; on the other hand, he could be said to have shown little basic improvement beyond slow maturation since admission. In October 1964 he was placed in the formal school class under a new woman teacher, as he had recently been showing some interest in learning in his play group.

Neville's remarkable sense of time was revealed by an incident at the end of the year. He was seen in the consulting-room by the writer and, on being asked how he was, replied that he had not been in the room for over a year, naming an actual day, which on checking indeed proved to be the last time he had been seen there. After making this point he lay on his back under the desk and carried on a conversation with the therapist from this position. The conversation was coherent and informed, recording the dates of several incidents in the unit, and including an account of his first visit to West Stowell.

After his Christmas leave Neville returned in a very unsettled mood and took almost a week to accept his houseparents again. At school he proved very difficult to handle, throwing water about, breaking equipment, and upsetting other children. His teacher was often obliged to return him to the House. When this happened Neville was very contrite, saying he would be a big boy now. By Easter he was staying at his desk for longer periods and could be persuaded to read and write simple words and attempt addition. He had a fair knowledge of numbers, largely retained from schooling before admission to West Stowell.

During the remainder of the year Neville showed definite signs of improvement and seemed to be benefiting from the demands made on him at school. His behaviour was slightly less obsessional and he could be relied on not to do any damage. This applied less at home, where he went through a long ritual of feeling all the walls of the house. Likewise, after being brought back to the unit he went through a fixed pattern of behaviour, looking at the clock, dashing off to the lavatory and urinating, after which he would lie on the floor and kick and laugh for a few minutes before dashing to the window to watch his father drive away.

At school he was happier now and doing more work. He tended to have fits of giggling, but stopped if told that his teacher could not be bothered with babies. He carried two sticks around with him much of the time, but could be persuaded to put them down and do some writing. His teacher felt that he had received a good grounding in writing and arithmetic and had good potential.

In September a new teacher came and Neville settled well with her. He was now ready to work and often seemed extra keen on doing sums in order to avoid contact with other members of the class, especially one boy of whom he was rather frightened. He showed good ability with sums and could read fluently from simple books. He wrote his name and could do simple sentences. When not given personal attention, he was happiest doing jigsaws or tracing routes on a road map of Wiltshire. He also enjoyed walks, and liked to guess the time they would reach various landmarks.

After Christmas he was transferred from the family group in which he was the oldest child to one that included other children of his own age. Here he seemed happier and sat on his own reading much of the time. In March 1966 he was tried at the local village school, at first on a part-time basis. He was very proud of this and coped well, although he was manifestly nervous. On one occasion in the trial period he had to be returned after wetting himself, urinating in the middle of the classroom. This was an isolated incident, and after Easter Neville attended full-time with little trouble. The head-master found him demanding, but willing to do sums with a little encouragement. For his age he was very retarded but seemed likely to make progress. His houseparents found that he was very anxious about going to school each morning but would be all right as long as they firmly insisted that he go. Neville now seemed to respond best to this, as if he appreciated certainty, whereas if kindly encouraged to do something he often refused or became silly and regressed to twitching and blinking. He remained an odd-looking child, very

175

emotional and restless, with an unusual speech pattern, but showing definite signs of stabilizing and making educational progress. His home remained a problem, as his behaviour appeared much worse there, and his parents were apparently resigned to this, refusing to deal with him firmly.

12. PAMELA

Born: 4 July 1956
Admitted: 17 June 1963
Reason for admission: gross conduct disorder in a severely deaf child; she had been excluded from a special school on the grounds that her problem was not deafness but conduct disorder
Height: 4 ft 1 in   Weight: 4 st 5 lb
IQ: 100+ (WISC)
EEG: not taken
Skull X-ray: refused to co-operate in being X-rayed
Bone-age: refused to co-operate in X-ray
Treatment: relationship therapy through child-centred intensive care; formal school class

Pamela's mother had always found her difficult to handle and had sent her to a special boarding school for the deaf at the age of $3\frac{1}{2}$. After three years she was excluded from this school because her behaviour indicated a primary conduct disorder rather than deafness. She was then sent to another special school where experience suggested emotional problems were more important than her deafness, and so she was referred to West Stowell.

Pamela's mother suffered from severe anaemia during pregnancy; the baby was three months premature and weighed only 2 lb 10 oz. It is reported that for the first twenty-five minutes after birth Pamela's lungs did not expand and oxygen was used. She was in an incubator for her first three months, and was fed by hand. At 2 days she had slight convulsions and was given calcium, after which she made a complete recovery. Later, while still in the incubator, she had mild pneumonia.

On returning from hospital at 3 months, Pamela weighed 5 lb 8 oz, and soon after this was officially diagnosed as deaf. At 4 months she was readmitted to hospital with pneumonia and received treatment for ten days. Her early milestones were anomalous. She sat up at 7 months, crawled at 9 months, but did not walk until 18 months. She showed a poor response to toilet-training. As a baby she liked to be rocked but showed little emotional response to her mother. As she grew older she became difficult to handle, and developed into an aggressive, obstinate, and overactive little girl.

At 2½ her mother brought her from Canada to England, where she thought better treatment facilities would be available. The journey was difficult, and Pamela's behaviour during it is described by her mother as 'like that of a wild animal'. After arrival she was seen by a specialist who recommended a boarding school for deaf children. Pamela went to one in October 1959 and stayed there as a boarder for the next three years. Her mother rejoined her husband abroad and both parents returned to England in 1960.

At boarding school Pamela's toilet habits regressed, and staff said she appeared to have no knowledge of how to use a pot. She was incontinent of urine and faeces, and generally wild and unsociable. She made contact with her teacher but not with other members of staff. During the first year her only contacts with her parents were letters and small presents sent to her every week. However, when her parents returned to England she began to go home for holidays, and some extra weekends. At about the same time she was taken out of a small school group and given individual teaching, which resulted in a new interest in learning, and better progress. Her behaviour remained a problem and she was emotionally highly reactive, especially with her mother. She refused to join in any group activities at school and became aggressive to any children who interfered with what she was doing. She was very severely deaf and responded only to the sound of loud fireworks or a burst balloon.

When Pamela was 6 her self-centred, contrary, and impulsive behaviour was presenting a major problem. An educational psychologist had been unable to gain her co-operation and expressed the belief that she was either defective or very disturbed. However, a later test, omitting verbal items, indicated that her ability was slightly above average, especially in shape discrimination.

When Pamela was excluded from school she was seen by a psychiatrist who suggested she might be suffering from an organically determined psychosis, the symptoms of which had been aggravated by

177

environmental factors. He saw her overactivity and distractibility as indicative of brain damage. Despite these views she was sent to another school for the deaf, attending from October 1962 when she was just over 6.

At this new school Pamela was described as an assertive and imaginative child of reasonable intelligence. She was very active and constantly gesturing in attempts to communicate. She could not lip-read, and would not respond to attempts to teach her. While at this school she attended a special unit for the deaf where she was not considered psychotic, and where her behaviour difficulties were thought to be largely reactive to the unsettling and bewildering experiences of being sent away to a boarding school at 3 following over-anxious management by her mother. Although she really needed to live at home, her mother, who suffered from severe psychosomatic ill health, was unable to accept Pamela's difficulties without more support than was available. In view of this, residential care was considered necessary, ideally offering treatment for her emotional problems.

Pamela was seen by the writer in May 1963, and admitted shortly after. Her mother said that she had never been an affectionate child, and had shown wilfulness from an early age. Toilet-training had been a battlefield; she would retain a motion and then pass it after leaving the toilet. Her mother told the writer she had herself been a premature baby, weighing only 2 lb 8 oz at birth and had been prone to ill-health in childhood. Pamela's father seemed very fond of his daughter and better able to control her than his wife. However, he played little part in her life and had withdrawn more and more into his work.

On admission Pamela gave the impression of being an intelligent, emotionally vulnerable child who was very uncertain in personal relationships but enjoyed affection. Her behaviour problems appeared mainly deprivational responses to three years in a boarding school when she was very young. Treatment was to consist of intensive relationships from all adults at all times, offered at as primary a level as she demanded. Every care was to be taken to minimize the frustrations liable to arise from her deafness. She was placed in the formal school group. Her parents were encouraged to visit as often as possible, and she was to go home for regular leaves.

Pamela, who was nearly 7 on admission, a well-built girl for her age, with brown hair and expressive brown eyes, was uneasy about her surroundings for the first few weeks, and wetted her bed most

178

nights. As her confidence built up, however, she emerged as a dominant figure in her family group. Her play was rough and boisterous, and she became excited very easily but proved quite amenable to warm, confident handling. Within a month of being admitted she was showing little of the self-centred, aggressive, and impulsive conduct that had previously made her unacceptable. She enjoyed attending school but failed to use her ability even to the extent her deafness allowed, because of emotional immaturity and contrariness when given tasks to complete. In August she spent a month at home. Her mother reported that she had not wet the bed at all, had seemed more settled, but still would not accept correction.

Over the rest of the year Pamela showed only occasional bouts of negativistic behaviour, often arising from frustration at her inability to express herself. She remained an excitable child but seemed to be controlling her aggression in the therapeutic environment at West Stowell. She began to take an interest in the other children and was protective towards Carol, a younger, fragile child. Pamela was so severely handicapped by her deafness that an ordinary hearing aid seemed to be of little use to her. The possibility of her really needing special schooling if her deafness was to be breached was constantly reviewed. However, the most important element was to stabilize her emotionally, and training as a deaf child was to be postponed until this had been achieved.

After a good home leave at Christmas, when her mother found her much less obstinate, Pamela returned to West Stowell to find the situation somewhat upset by a number of staff changes.

In spring 1964 the atmosphere restabilized with the arrival of new houseparents and a new teacher. Treatment now returned to intensive measures to build up her ability to make relationships with adults. Her new houseparents found her excitable and often aggressive. Attempts to communicate through facial expression did not succeed, and a different approach was used, concentrating on physical contact and imitating, combined with carefully mouthed words. Pamela responded well to this. Much of her extreme excitement and aggression fell away and seemed to be replaced by determined efforts to make contact. As her houseparents began to communicate more with her, she seemed to become calmer and more co-operative with them. Care had to be taken to avoid situations that were much beyond her capacity, as she could seldom control herself and would

179

end up in a frenzied state with prolonged high-pitched screaming accompanied by violence towards people and things.

The new teacher, a married woman with children of Pamela's age, was able to get a very good response from her. After some initial tantrums she responded to a fairly demanding approach. By the middle of the year her teacher found it possible to communicate by simple phrases written down. Pamela showed interest in numbers but made little attempt to work with them herself. She was not at all responsive to attempts to make her follow lip movements, and in other fields was rather resentful of instruction or correction. Her teacher, however, felt she had made good progress, especially as the other children made little allowance for her deafness.

Pamela's summer leave reflected her general improvement. The only incident reminiscent of former behaviour was when she had a tantrum in the street outside a shop because her mother refused to buy her a bicycle.

Over the rest of the year Pamela's forceful attention-seeking diminished. The bouts of hysterical screaming became rare. She had become one of the more affectionate children in the unit, but still needed much attention, particularly affectionate physical contact.

During 1965 Pamela continued to mature. She was becoming a useful member of her family group and helped with the younger children. She was less impulsive, and much happier in the assurance that she could communicate with her houseparents by gestures and sounds. At school she worked with the other children, and by the time she went on leave in August had reached the stage of doing simple addition, subtraction, and multiplication. She could copy efficiently and relate single words to pictures. It was felt that she required specialized teaching more, now that emotional stability and social competence were being achieved. Ideally she needed a unit for deaf children with emotional problems. Piecemeal training from a speech therapist or peripatetic special teacher who would not have time to build a relationship with her was unlikely to succeed.

At home in the summer her main difficulty lay in her relationship with her mother, who said that Pamela responded only to corporal punishment as a means of correction. Before this she had scratched and bitten her mother when corrected. Following return to West Stowell Pamela showed no evidence of emotional difficulties or disturbed behaviour.

Pamela's teacher had left in July, but she made an equally good relationship with a new teacher who came in September, and continued to make good progress. She was now 9 years old. In the next two terms she extended her abilities so that she could add and subtract hundreds, tens, and units, multiply and divide, and match short sentences to relevant pictures. It was still hard to get her to concentrate for very long, and she was liable to walk round the classroom after a successful bit of work. She was not difficult to control, however, and showed no aggression except retaliation against other children's attacks. She was much more willing to accept instruction in class, and, in co-operation with the responsible local authority, steps were taken to provide exceptionally powerful hearing equipment to help the teacher communicate with her.

At Christmas 1965 and Easter 1966 Pamela was better at home. Her mother found her able to accept correction and described the holiday in eulogistic terms. At West Stowell House she presented no real problems. She was a happy child, who greeted all staff she knew with a boisterous hug and kiss. She still tended to be rather rough with smaller children and would drag back to his or her room any child who ran off, announcing the misdemeanour with a string of indignant noises.

Pamela remained a highly reactive child. Although she became very excited at other children's behaviour and retaliated strongly if attacked, generally she was stable and conformative in the context of West Stowell House. On a school trip to a fire station she became frightened when a fire-engine was moved as a demonstration, pushing her teacher to the wall and pointing out worriedly that she might be run over. Misinterpretation of situations, leading to excessive nervousness, often seemed to be the basis of her aggression, contrariness, and tantrums.

By May 1966 Pamela was nearly 10 and had been in the unit for three years. She had responded well to the child-centred intensive care, especially in her family group, and had benefited from an educational approach that made allowances for her emotional problems as well as her deafness. She was still very responsive but could now maintain stability and make good progress provided her environment was an accepting one. Successful home leaves suggested that she was beginning to make a better adjustment to her mother. It was still necessary to avoid a situation whereby Pamela was treated as an emotionally stable deaf child, but it was expected that she would be ready to leave West Stowell within the next year, provided that her new placement recognized her special emotional problems. The prognosis seemed good.

13. PAUL

Born: 27 July 1957
Admitted: 21 February 1961
Discharged: 8 January 1965
Reason for admission: autistic child with motor action suggestive of brain damage
Height: 3 ft   Weight: 2 st 7 lb
IQ: untestable
EEG: not taken
Skull X-ray: normal
Bone-age: 4 years when 4
Treatment: Regressed nurtural care, with additional individual nursing

Paul was referred to West Stowell House from another hospital where he had been described as mute and autistic, with apparent sensory imperception. He had had a very disturbed childhood, and his parents were separated.

His birth was difficult and prolonged and required forceps delivery. He weighed 10 lb and needed an oxygen tent. After two weeks in hospital he went home, was breast-fed for four weeks, and then placed on the bottle.

From the start Paul was not looked after by his mother but by an old nanny who had looked after his father when *he* was a baby. He seemed very contented. On being questioned much later, his mother said that at no time, even in earliest infancy, had Paul been able to make the outgoing easy contact that is normally achieved between baby and mother.

Most of Paul's development in the first year was within normal limits. He sat up at 8 months and was walking by 14 months. However, he would never sit on a potty. His nanny would tie him to it, and he would cry whenever she said 'Come and sit on the potty'. He started to regurgitate from an early age, possibly as a result of excessive feeding. By the time he was 1 year old he was showing enjoyment in a number of activities, especially watching television and being dressed up in his mother's clothes.

During his first year the family moved twice, and his mother saw less and less of Paul. She was described as 'unstable, ambitious, and extravagant' and was said to drink heavily. Father seems to have played only a minimal role in Paul's early life. Reports describe him as 'highly intelligent but anti-social'. He became very angry whenever the child cried and seemed to have a general dislike of him. The nanny, who had more contact than anyone else with Paul in these early years, seems to have been at once domineering and very over-protective.

Photographs taken of Paul at 15 months show an apparently normal child, but his grandparents recalled that at this time he had long periods when he would take no notice of anything going on around him, and would run round apparently vacantly and purposelessly. When he was 18 months old he began to wake weeping during the night, and on most nights his nanny had to get up to comfort him, often taking him to her room until he slept again.

By the time he was 2 years old little speech had developed. He said 'Hello' and 'Bye-bye' but nothing else. His difficulty here may be partly attributable to the fact that his nanny spoke to him only in a foreign language. From this time on he became more manifestly abnormal. He seemed frequently to fall and on one occasion fell down the stairs badly, though no physical damage apparently occurred. He became very angry if he saw his nanny nursing his sister and also if he saw his mother and father embracing. Many other things, such as the dismantling of his playpen, could easily upset him.

Paul had still shown no response to toilet-training. He made little attempt to do anything for himself and had to be dressed, washed, and fed. If a door did not open at once he would run away rather than try again to open it himself. Most of the time he wandered about restlessly with a clumsy gait. He ate anything he came across, appropriate or not, and mouthed large objects.

When he was 2½ Paul's parents separated. Retrospectively, it has not been possible to ascertain for how long the home background had been grossly disturbing and emotionally damaged. In May 1960, when he was nearly 3 years old, Paul's nanny also left, and the steady deterioration in his condition continued. He did not take to any of her successors, and most left quickly, finding him impossible to cope with. He soiled continuously, had taken to eating and smearing his faeces, and was almost totally withdrawn. His mother found it impossible to cope with him on her own, and in December 1960 he was admitted to hospital. He showed no reaction to auditory and other sensory stimuli, although his peripheral sensory system was intact. Shortly before this he had been seen by a consultant children's psychiatrist, who thought he was autistic but also intrinsically backward, and attributed his withdrawn and disturbed condition to the impact of the loss of his nanny on a very vulnerable child.

It was felt that Paul was in need of intensive psychotherapeutic treatment if he were to recover at all, and he was, therefore, referred to West Stowell House, where he was admitted shortly after. At this stage one of the most notable features in his condition was his shambling, staggering gait and general difficulty with co-ordination. His mouth hung open, with his face in a grimace. At times he seemed to come into contact with his environment for short periods, glancing about in an alert interested manner, and at such moments his gait was normal, but the general pattern of behaviour gave the impression of a psychotic self-absorption with very minor outgoing traits, which was equivalent to severe subnormality and might be associated with it. It was hard to decide how far his behaviour was reactive and how much the result of a basically vulnerable personality, associated with possible progressive brain damage. At times his condition appeared to be severe subnormality with a few psychotic features; at others his lack of contact seemed chosen and deliberate.

Paul was placed in a therapeutic play group where he would receive regressed nurtural care. In addition to this, he was given considerable individual nursing aimed at building up a reliable, primitive relationship with an adult. He was always put to bed individually, as far as possible by the same person on all occasions. At first he would not even walk and had to be taken round the unit in a pram. When given a baby's bottle he did not suck and he would not respond to cuddling. Staff commented on him as the most withdrawn child they had ever known.

Nothing was seen of his parents, but his grandparents visited regularly and showed great interest in Paul. At first he was un-interested in their visits and quite out of touch, but during a visit in April, two months after admission, he made a transient affectionate dependent relationship with them. He also seemed to be developing episodic relationships with staff. In therapeutic sessions he would edge into the room in an evasive manner and avoid looking directly at the therapist, although he seemed to watch when he thought he was not being observed. In the unit he was reported as being in and out of touch all the time. He had the habit of putting objects in his mouth, including gravel, grass, and toys. Because of his overactivity he received a sedative at night on a routine basis for a period.

In the latter half of the year he made no progress. He would still do nothing for himself and became increasingly miserable and de-pressed, weeping for no reason and lying half-curled up in a corner, taking no notice of anyone. A course of tranquillizers was tried to see if it would help him, but later the drug was withdrawn as it seemed to make him drowsy much of the time.

From admission, Paul had been in a family group. His house-parents said he was ignoring them less after a few months. By the end of the year he was accepting toilet control but taking no re-sponsibility for it. He had begun to feed himself with a little dry food at meals but usually dropped a cup if given one. In his play group he lolled about on the floor looking for something to put into his mouth, and showing little interest in, or awareness of, the world around him. Towards the end of the year his regurgitations returned and he began to indulge in anal play. He staggered about the unit in a grotesque hypotonic manner, his head hanging down on one side, with little contact with staff or fellow-patients. After a year in West Stowell he had made scarcely any improvement beyond the slight progress noted in the first few months.

During 1962 he appeared more and more as if he were a severely subnormal child of very limited contact. A course of nico-tinomide was tried but did not appear to have any effect. At times he seemed to be making small moves forward, in terms of relationships and contact, but when seen in retrospect at the end of the year these seemed minimal. He would stay clinging to his play therapist for longer periods and appeared to enjoy being nursed, but showed no expansion of interest. He liked to climb and run about and would often do this rather than lie on the floor and mouth objects as he

185

had done at first. His houseparents thought he was happier and more aware of the reactions of adults. They also found him a little more co-operative over being dressed. The general feeling by the end of the year was that there had been a quantitative decrease in his grossly abnormal behaviour, but no change in its basic pattern.

Paul was now 5½. During 1963 his condition showed little change. In some respects he seemed to be getting worse, and there was more smearing and soiling. He sucked his thumb most of the time in an aggressive manner, often until it was raw, and ate dirt and faeces whenever he had the opportunity. He still had to be fed, and his conduct in general was unpredictable. He would collapse onto the ground if involved in anything in which he did not wish to participate, and seemed resentful of other children. In his therapeutic play group he was as far as ever from constructive play, spending his time in dashing round, thumb in mouth, knocking toys off tables. His houseparents felt that by the end of the year, when they had had him for over two years, he had made some progress. They commented that his withdrawal seemed deliberate and self-chosen. This attitude had also been noticed by the writer during psychotherapeutic sessions, when Paul often seemed to be watching and summing up the therapist while maintaining his withdrawal.

By August 1964 Paul had been in the unit for three and a half years. He was 7. The apparently wilful withdrawal continued, and it was noted that his awareness seemed to increase only in a relationship with one of the domestics who had become very fond of him. Otherwise neither his play therapist nor his houseparents had noticed any progress for some time. He remained incontinent of both urine and faeces and had shown no signs of any constructive play or real contact with adults. He had not responded to treatment at an intensive level and though it was still felt that Paul was not a stable, severely subnormal child, there was no indication that he could respond to a therapeutic approach better than to long-term training. In view of this he was transferred to the boys' ward at Pewsey Hospital in January 1965.

On follow-up in May 1966, Paul, now nearly 9 years old, was still at Pewsey Hospital, and there had been no progress in his development.

14. RICHARD

Born: 4 September 1960

Admitted: 3 May 1965

Reason for admission: Juvenile psychosis; hyperkinetic and with-drawn. Referred from children's hospital

Height: 3 ft 5½ in   Weight: 3 st

IQ: untestable

EEG: Diffuse abnormality with slight asymmetry between the activity of the two hemispheres

Skull X-ray: X-ray normal; head circumference above average size for age

Bone-age: *c.* 3½ at 5 years.

Treatment: regressed nurtural care in play group

Richard was the first child of normal healthy parents. Pregnancy and confinement were normal and he weighed 7 lb 3 oz at birth. His mother's milk failed, so he was bottle-fed from the sixth day. From 2 months onwards he was left with the bottle and seems never to have been nursed by his mother. Toilet-training was strict from an early date but he never responded properly.

Richard sat up at 7 months, crawled at 10 months and walked when a year old. By 18 months he had a number of words and would count 'one, two, three'. By this time he was also feeding himself with a spoon. He did not sleep very well and was taken to the family doctor because of this. He assessed Richard as a normally developing child of a rather apprehensive mother. Shortly after his second birthday the family moved house, and his mother began to prepare for her second child, who was born when Richard was 2 years 5 months.

Richard's difficulties seem to date from this period. His speech made no progress, and in fact got worse. He refused even to try to dress himself, and developed a number of mannerisms; he mouthed objects, tapped surfaces, and like to flick his fingers. At the same time he became withdrawn and overactive, jealous and stubborn. He resisted any contact with his sister, and refused to go near his parents if she were with them. More and more he refused affection and seemed to have no interest in his environment. He was seen again by his general practitioner, who now found him overactive and obsessional.

At the age of 4 he went into a children's hospital for a period of three weeks' observation. According to his father, he was in a cot restrainer all the time he was there. His withdrawal and repetitive behaviour were thought to indicate a psychotic condition. Attempts to assess his intelligence failed. He was sent home without any recommended treatment other than a request for admission to West Stowell House.

Richard was brought for interview by his parents when he was 4½, and was quite content to be taken away to play elsewhere in the unit after a short time. During the interview his behaviour had been restless and manneristic. He moved away squealing when approached, and, if left, covered his ears and flicked his fingers. His mother commented on his habit of carrying round two wooden bricks which he would manipulate, clapping them together, altering surfaces, usually in mid-air, but also on a flat surface such as a table.

Richard's mother lacked confidence in her handling of him and admitted that she had been very uncertain as to how to bring him up. Her husband, a semi-skilled manual worker, appeared to be a spontaneous, straightforward man. Their second child, a 2-year-old girl, was a pleasant, happy child and their attitude towards her seemed normal and loving. They seemed ready to admit mistakes in their early handling of Richard, and were prepared to participate in any way they could to help him.

Richard was assessed as an autistic child whose mental retardation seemed secondary to his emotional disturbance. Though there were reactive elements, investigation was thought likely to reveal organic features.

On admission Richard was upset by the new routine, but soon settled and accepted his surroundings with apparent placidity and a certain detachment. His mother stayed nearby for a few days to help him settle in.

Richard could not speak but drew attention to himself by physical gesture. By day he was clean, if caught; at night he needed raising. He ate with spoon and fingers, but had to be washed, dressed, and undressed. He was placed in a therapeutic play group and a family group, but showed little contact with adults and less with children.

In the first weeks Richard regressed, becoming more infantile and dependent, and it was decided to make use of this to bring him through a secondary infancy. With a view to this he was moved into the therapeutic play group consisting of less outgoing children, and transferred to a family group of younger children.

In his play group Richard's psychotic mannerisms were soon observed. His play was unconstructive, and he was happiest climbing on the mantelpiece or lying on his stomach babbling to himself. He carried two bricks around with him and would sit clapping these together. They seemed to act as security symbols for him. He seemed very sensitive to noise, and would cover his ears if there was too much, or any sudden, noise.

When first interviewed in the consulting-room Richard seemed very upset at being moved from his play group. He seemed to live in a world of his own, making only occasional transient contact with the writer. He generally showed little interest in adults but responded to his mother when she visited. It was felt that Richard could be helped, and his trial admission was extended to at least a year.

In June Richard was visited by his grandparents. His initial reaction was to shrink away, whining, but he was persuaded to go out for a walk with them. He reacted similarly a few weeks later when visited by his parents. On the other hand, he was beginning to show some signs of emotional satisfaction from adult embraces, when he could be brought into contact. However, for much of the time he seemed to be preoccupied with his own inner life; at meals he would often sit leaning his head on his elbows with his hands clasped over his ears, making no response to overtures from adults or the offer of food or comforting.

After a successful home leave, during which his parents found him much happier and more affectionate, Richard began to move forward a little at West Stowell, responding briefly to the approaches of his play therapist, and answering his name if called. In the consulting-room he often seemed resentful and negativistic, but this seemed a possible advance on his previous withdrawn attitude. He continued to be resistant to change and still did not like being brought from his play group to the consulting-room. He was less anxious and depressed, but his clapping together of objects persisted, though he was not quite so obsessively attached to the bricks he used to carry round with him. The mouthing of objects and scratching of surfaces had virtually disappeared by the end of the year, and there was a general softening of his obsessional anxiety. An EEG revealed a continuing minor diffuse abnormality.

o

By the beginning of 1966, when Richard had been in the unit for seven months, his progress had been slower than originally hoped but there were definite signs of a response to affection, and his anxiety was now little more than watchfulness. Much of his manneristic behaviour persisted; he waved his hands in front of his eyes and played much of the time with his two bricks. However, these traits seemed less compulsive. There were no signs of speech re-emerging, but he did say 'Mum' and 'Dad' frequently. Though still living in his own world, with little contact with adults, he was not so determinedly withdrawn, and no longer resisted affection.

At Easter 1966 his parents reported a noticeable improvement. There were more attempts at communicating and he showed a friendly, interested approach to his sister. At West Stowell this was paralleled by a spontaneous relationship he had built up with another autistic child. The two would romp together, obviously affording each other much pleasure. On one occasion, when the other boy was ill, Richard was clearly puzzled at the lack of response in his former playmate. This attitude did not extend to other children, of whom he seemed rather apprehensive. He was now much more prepared to make contact with adults and only reverted to his hand-waving and brick-playing when upset. His parents seemed to have more confidence in handling him, and it was felt that he should eventually be able to go home. He is likely to continue on a retarded level but was showing signs of response to regressed nurtural care. There seemed good reason to expect that after a further year or so he would be able to progress to some form of schooling within the unit.

15. ROGER

Born: 20 July 1953
Admitted: 10 October 1958
Discharged: 2 April 1966
Reason for admission: Overactive manneristic behaviour; admitted for observation as possible psychosis
Height: 3 ft 6 in   Weight: 3 st
IQ: untestable
EEG: epileptic focus in left temporal region, 1965

Skull X-ray: normal; circumference large as a child

Bone-age: *c.* 5 years when 8

Treatment: Child-centred intensive care; family group 1961 onwards
   September 1959–September 1964: regressed nurtural care in
      therapeutic play group with short periods in nursery-school class
   September 1964–April 1966: Froebel nursery class

Roger was referred to West Stowell House by a local health deparment that felt uncertain about diagnosis and requested a period of in-patient observation. He had been attending day nursery where his behaviour had been withdrawn and manneristic.

No details are available about Roger's birth and early development. His mother said that although he had been backward from birth, she thought the birth was normal. However, many of her observations were inconsistent.

Roger's father deserted soon after his conception, and the child and his mother lived in one room for his first four years. His mother had to go to work to support them, and Roger was at first looked after by a series of baby-minders during the day, and later placed in a day nursery at 13 months for mornings only. At 2 years he was not using sounds to communicate and had shown no response to toilet-training. He was overactive and appeared unable to relate to his mother or to anyone else.

At the day nursery he needed constant attention, running away or destroying toys if not watched closely. He was very withdrawn, and the staff found it impossible to make any normal contact with him. He was referred to hospital for observation, but no definite diagnosis seems to have been made, and Roger continued to live at home and attend the nursery.

In March 1957, when nearly 4, Roger again was referred to hospital and diagnosed as suffering from a hyperkinetic syndrome of unknown aetiology. Attempts to assess his intelligence failed because of his overactive behaviour. There appeared to be no abnormality in the central nervous system.

Roger still lived with his mother in a single room where conditions were described as 'very poor indeed'. They shared a bed and general sanitary conditions were very inadequate. His mother was working full-time and seemed unable to cope with his excessive behaviour, especially as she was usually tired after work. She alternated between indulging him and hitting him, and had little idea of how to handle him, though she appeared very fond of him.

At the nursery Roger's behaviour did not change, and in June 1958, at the matron's request, he was examined by a doctor who remarked on his aloofness and lack of interest in the other children's activities. The doctor thought Roger less overactive than earlier reports suggested, and found him able to respond to simple commands. He thought rudimentary speech sounds and other behaviour suggested a psychosis rather than simple mental defect. At the nursery he had no contact with the other children and preferred to sit alone playing with pieces of paper, which he tore into strips or folded over at the corners in a stereotyped manner. He always smelled sweets before eating them and would often approach a person by smelling rather than smiling or uttering. For the past year Roger had been regularly attending a speech clinic at a children's hospital where it had been noticed that he was making some progress towards speech and that his restlessness was decreasing. In August he was seen by a consultant children's psychiatrist, who agreed that he was displaying psychotic behaviour. A longer period of observation would be needed before diagnostic differentiation between the effects of early emotional deprivation, subnormality, and a possible psychosis could be made.

Roger was brought to West Stowell by his mother, a small almost dwarfish woman with a bustling extraverted attitude. She was simple and unaffected and rather uncertain about her attitude towards Roger. Soon after his admission she remarried, but within a year the marriage broke up.

On admission Roger was a normal-looking boy of average build with brown hair and blue eyes and a habit of suddenly grimacing for no apparent reason. He had no speech, could not dress or undress himself, was incontinent and a messy feeder. When his mother left he cried disconsolately at first but after a few hours settled and did not appear to miss her. He was very overactive and frequently aggressive towards other children, causing minor injuries to them on a number of occasions. Though withdrawn and out of contact for much of the time, he often appeared happy and could be heard singing quietly to himself. Apart from this he derived most pleasure from simple repetitive activities such as paper-tearing, sweeping dust off the floor, and wandering in the gardens picking up objects and sniffing them.

In October 1959, when the reorganization of the unit began, Roger was 6 years old and had been at West Stowell for a year. He was still incontinent and unable to dress, but his eating habits were less messy. He had a considerable number of food fads and would always smell his food before eating it. He was inclined to wander off unless carefully watched when in the garden. Verbalizing was poor, limited, and not used for communicating, but if encouraged he was able to repeat most of the better known nursery rhymes, singing them in a badly articulated but rhythmical manner. His behaviour confirmed the earlier diagnosis of a severely disturbed, psychotic child. Management was concentrated on attempts to establish relationships with him, keeping him in physical contact as far as possible, and not allowing him to wander away or withdraw into himself. He received regular psychotherapy from the writer. In these sessions he avoided face-to-face situations and would go through elaborate rituals of slowly developing contact.

In the first few months of 1960 small advances were noticed in his capacity for relationships. He would occasionally smile at staff and there were fleeting forerunners of spontaneous speech, especially when he was alone with an adult. One member of staff encouraged Roger to come up to his flat, where Roger began to repeat an occasional word and also ate meals far more tidily than when he was with other children. Often, however, he still ignored approaches, concentrating – in a dreamy way – on his paper-tearing. He enjoyed walks in the country with one of the staff but otherwise remained withdrawn. In his play group he showed only manneristic repetitive play. This pattern of behaviour continued until the middle of the year, when it was decided that a more intensive approach would be needed to make useful contact with him.

Roger's mother had proved unable to take any active role in his treatment, since she lived in the North of England and had no room to take him for leaves. It was, therefore, decided to place him and two other children with a single member of staff whom they had all known for some time, who would spend most of her time with them encouraging talk, constructive play, and simple relationships. After a month he made enough contact with the other children to be able to share play with a toy. He also began to make spontaneous approaches to the play therapist, climbing on her lap and clearly enjoying physical contact. His echolalia now had an element of learning, in that it reflected interest in certain phrases and their appropriate use. One further indication of the success of this move was that by the end of the year his soiling had diminished considerably. He had also begun to take an interest in self-imposed tasks such as solving jigsaws, and became upset when he could not complete these. He still showed little interest in other children, but aggression towards them was becoming rarer. The main advance was in his need for a relationship with adults, which he now sought of his own accord.

At the beginning of January 1961 the play therapist in charge of Roger's small group left. He showed marked regression with some withdrawal, overactivity, hostility, and lack of toilet-control. By April he had recovered the position reached before his therapist left; soiling had ceased and he was making spontaneous approaches to adults. Even during his period of regression the aggressive and disinterested behaviour displayed when he first came to West Stowell had not reappeared.

Roger was now in a larger play group with a new therapist. He spent most of his time alone doing jigsaws, at which he showed considerable ability. Other activities included tearing books into strips and climbing on top of cupboards. His therapist felt he was the most able child in her group, though very backward. He learned to repeat multiplication tables up to four but did not respond to attempts to interest him in pre-reading activities. Speech was increasing, but he still tended only to repeat words and phrases. He could recite the alphabet and knew the names of all members of staff and of the other children in the unit.

In June Roger was placed in a family group in the care of two houseparents. Although he still preferred to be alone, he had been showing more interest in tentative relationships with adults and now developed these within the intimate atmosphere of his group. By the end of 1961 he was enjoying sitting on his housemother's knee and could carry out simple conversations with her and ask for a kiss. He had learned a number of new songs from the radio and enjoyed singing these without words. In the garden he displayed remarkable climbing ability, but in most respects his level of performance remained severely retarded, around the 4-year-old level. His mother had visited on several occasions, on the last of which Roger had run up to her and called her 'Mummy', where previously he had always sidled up and said 'Hello Mrs Smith' or 'Say good-bye to Mrs Smith'.

Roger continued to have regular psychotherapeutic sessions with the writer. When these had first started in 1959 he evaded contact by hiding under a table or chair and refusing all approaches. After some months he would emerge at the end of a session and approach the desk and even sit on the therapist's knee. Then gradually the elaborate ritual was shortened and by the end of 1960 he would establish contact without first lying on the floor and wriggling all round the room. Even so, conversations often had to be carried out with Roger sitting under a table or turning his back on the therapist. For a long time these 'conversations' were purely echolalic. The writer would say 'Have a sweet, Roger', and Roger would echo these words. The breakthrough came after nearly two years, when Roger first answered such an offer of a sweet with 'Yes', rather than a repetition. He seemed very embarrassed and confused at having done this. Later he developed a number of spontaneous phrases and would address the writer by name. His speech for a long time remained predominantly echolalic, but he began to make spontaneous use of echoed phrases and used names appropriately. Face-to-face confrontation was, however, still a very difficult thing for him and he tended to speak at the ground rather than directly.

Roger still soiled once or twice a week, but there had been no return of the deliberate soiling that had marked his period of regression at the beginning of the year. Over the rest of the year he continued to improve, and in view of this, and the fact that he was talking a lot more, it was decided that he should be tried in the nursery-school class.

In the first few months of 1962 Roger continued to make good progress. At school he proved resistant to teaching, and it was felt that some months might have to elapse before he accepted the classroom situation. In late spring his housemother left suddenly, and Roger was clearly affected by this and showed signs of regression in the unit and in school. He soiled regularly at school, and smeared his bed. To ease the situation, he was transferred to a therapeutic play group where he would return to primary relationship-making. Routine toileting was also restarted. These measures slowly led to a return of emotional control and imposed social competence.

In September 1962, when he was 9, new houseparents took over his family group. He adapted to them well, and it was felt that he was now ready to start school again. It soon became apparent, however, that Roger was still some way from learning to read and

195

do arithmetic and he was changed to the nursery class, where he was far happier. His houseparents found him willing to converse in an indirect question-and-answer way, but said that he was often very withdrawn. He enjoyed the Music and Movement sessions and any opportunity to listen and sing to music. Staff changes during the year had affected him, as his difficulties with relationships seemed to outweigh the other elements in his severe handicap.

Over the next year Roger's progress continued. He was making better contact with his houseparents, and would approach strangers in the unit, making contact by means of a ritual of naming parts of the body. He would ask 'Where's your nose?' 'Where's your mouth?' and get apparent satisfaction from the responses, although he did not seem particularly disturbed if these were incorrect. At school for a long time he would attempt nothing. If teased by other children, he became very angry and would bump his head on the wall or desk. His favourite activity was listening to music. If pressed hard enough he would occasionally match and sort shapes, but he generally disliked most things he was asked to do. Towards the end of the year he became restless, annoying other children and breaking pieces of equipment. He refused to do jigsaws which had previously been a favourite pastime and broke up other puzzles. In November his teacher left, and he returned to a therapeutic play group where his behaviour was less aggressive, but where he still did little. He went through his ritual of naming parts of the body with his play therapist every morning, after which he would sit on her lap for a while before moving away to be on his own.

By the beginning of 1964 Roger had been in the unit for over four years and was $10\frac{1}{2}$ years old. In this time he had never been back to his home and had had fewer visits than most children. He seemed likely to be suffering from prolonged institutionalization, and arrangements were made for him to stay at a boys' hostel at Easter, while his mother lived nearby and took him out by the day. He was well-behaved during this fortnight and, though he would not mix with other children, played happily with books and jigsaws.

This contrasted with the much more disturbed behaviour Roger showed at West Stowell in the first few months of 1964. He was more aggressive towards younger children, biting them and being bitten in return. He also seemed more anxious, constantly asking the time, and coming in and out of contact when talking to people.

In summer he again went to the hostel, during which period his mother said he was better in all respects, apart from toilet habits, which were still unreliable. He continued in his play group for most of the year, but in September 1964 started in a new nursery-school group, in which he settled very well. He enjoyed school and was always first there to greet his teacher; 'There's Miss X. Had a good dinner? Enjoy your fish and chips?' His teacher commented that his mannerisms persisted; and he almost stripped the room of wallpaper. He was easily demoralized by any change of pattern and routine, responding to such occurrences by singing a familiar nursery rhyme, or going through his naming-of-parts ritual. He was developing a predilection for collecting and eating food from the refuse and pig bins.

In May 1964 new houseparents had taken over his family group, the previous ones having left in November 1963. They found Roger very difficult to make contact with. He never initiated play as other children in the group did, and often appeared quite out of contact. Towards the end of 1964 he began to have 'sleepy spells' which later were seen as *petit mal* seizures. One morning his face was noticed to be flaccid, his eyes staring, and his body slumped in a sitting position. He remained like this for five minutes, during which he made no response to stimulation.

At Christmas 1964 Roger went home, this time staying with his mother, and not at the hostel. The leave was a satisfactory one, though his mother said he was wet on a number of occasions. She had requested that he be moved nearer to her, and it was hoped that in the next year or so he might be able to improve to the point of being transferred to a hostel from which he could attend a training centre.

At school Roger was achieving little educationally, but showed ability at matching shapes, colours, and numbers. He had a keen eye for detail, which seemed to be the positive side of his obsessive desire for sameness. At first he was unable to draw a circle, square, or triangle so as to differentiate them, but he learned to do so after his teacher made him trace their outline with his finger, and later this approach helped in teaching him letters. He was now often sent back to the House at playtime, because of his compulsive ferreting in dustbins, which ended in his eating whatever he found. In February he had another fit, in which he suddenly appeared dazed and pallid and slumped forward in his chair, yawning and closing his eyes, after which he slept for about fifteen minutes. A similar attack occurred in the next month. His teacher noticed that Roger had recently started masturbating; he would ask to go to the toilet and then later she would find him in the kitchen with his trousers down, having produced an erection. He did not do this in public, either at school or in his family group.

After a successful home leave in April 1965 Roger had a number of further ictal attacks over the next few months. These were becoming more frequent, and treatment was started. An EEG revealed an epileptic focus, mainly in the left temporal region.

At school Roger had responded to attempts by his teacher to make use of his interest in shapes and surfaces by a tactile approach to letters. Though nearly 12 he had no knowledge of letters and had shown little interest in them. He did, however, manage jigsaws and shape-matching. His teacher first persuaded him to trace letters and then to match plastic-shaped letters when he could feel as well as see differences. Later she made use of large wooden letters and letters made out of sandpaper stuck on cardboard. By the end of the year he had learned to copy out the letters of the alphabet. He made some small moves beyond this, learning to match a few words against their relevant pictures and to read and write his name. He could also write several letters if asked to by his teacher.

Because of his epileptic condition and the unsatisfactory home circumstances, Roger did not go away from West Stowell in the summer. He seemed very conscious of this and talked constantly of 'Going up to Liverpool to see Mrs Smith'. He was still being treated with small doses of mysoline and epanutin but in September suffered two further *petit mal* attacks after each of which he slept for periods of twenty or thirty minutes. Finally, in late October, he had a *grand mal* attack. Alongside this worsening of his epileptic condition, Roger's behaviour became more aggressive. He bit other children in his class if they upset him, and his mood was generally irritable and uneasy. He was masturbating more frequently and at the age of 12 seemed now to be facing the additional problems of puberty and awakening of sexual awareness.

He received increased doses of anti-convulsant drugs and these controlled his attacks, but he remained in a generally sullen and dejected mood. At a West Stowell House party held in November he

198

showed no response at all, scarcely aware of what was going on. Towards the end of the year he brightened up, and began to take an interest in people, giving a running commentary on all who passed by his school window, and calling out greetings to those he knew well. However, his overall position now seemed fairly stationary and he did not show the potential that had been noticed a year or so earlier.

At Christmas he went to stay with his mother and enjoyed a good leave, during which he had only one mild fit. Just before he went on leave Roger's houseparents left and his teacher went on prolonged sick leave. This meant that on return the usual pattern of his day had altered and this seemed to have a disturbing effect on him. He began to show acts of impulsive aggression, hitting out at other children or suddenly pulling their hair with no provocation. He was also becoming destructive, tearing up table cloths and his bedroom curtains, and throwing things out of the window. He had to be moved from the bedroom he was sharing with some relatively small boys, because of a tendency to get into bed with them. Roger now showed little interest in the life of the unit and spent most of his time alone, lying on the floor or on the mantelpiece in one of the family-group rooms. He improved slightly when his teacher returned, and became quite skilful at a toy zither which he could play by following a patterned tune. However, it was becoming apparent that he had reached the limit of what could be done for him and arrangements were made for his return to the North. He was discharged to his home in April 1966 prior to admission to a hospital for the subnormal where his mother could more readily keep in contact with him.

16. ROY

Born: 6 April 1957

Admitted: 22 January 1962

Reason for admission: infantile autism; mother was admitted to a mental hospital and the children's home to which Roy was sent could not cope with so disturbed a child

Height: 3 ft 4 in   Weight: 3 st

IQ: untestable

EEG: normal

Skull X-ray: normal, but circumference smaller than average
Bone-age: 4 years when 5
Treatment: regressed nurtural care in therapeutic play group
   child-centred intensive care in family group
   April 1966: mornings only in formal school class

Roy came to West Stowell as an emergency case after his mother had been admitted to a mental hospital. He was staying temporarily at a children's home, as his father was in the services and so could not look after him. At the home he was aggressive towards the younger children and was felt to be a potential danger to them. He had been diagnosed at the age of 3 as having 'a genuine Kannerian psychosis'.

Roy was the third child of his mother, who was then 22. He was an unplanned child. Labour was difficult and he weighed 9 lb 1 oz. He was reported as an exceptionally healthy and attractive infant, and was breast-fed until 5 months, after which he was weaned easily. He always fed and slept well. He sat up at 7 months, crawled at 8 months and walked at 16 months. He is said to have been toilet-trained by 10 months. His mother said he was a very loving child towards people he knew, and very demanding of affection and cuddling. She described him as 'sitting on my lap with legs either side of me and rocking back and forward'. In retrospect, Roy's actions suggest he may have been essentially a symbiotic child using his mother as a cuddling-machine.

Although he liked to rock as an infant and was described as 'dreamy', Roy also seems to have shown a lively interest in his surroundings during his first year, and played with boxes, bricks, and other objects in a fairly constructive way. However, his parents noticed that he was 'unusual', especially towards other children, as from the age of 1 year they had to keep him away from them in case he hit them. On the other hand, he was said to have played well with his two older brothers. In all the circumstances, it was difficult to judge how far his mother's account of Roy's early life was reliable, as she seemed to remember him as an exceptionally superior child.

At 18 months Roy could say a few words, but later he suddenly stopped talking altogether. He grew increasingly inquisitive, and this resulted in his also being destructive in an investigatory way. His parents were living abroad, and when Roy was 2 they moved into a new house, which disturbed him. At first he refused to go into it, and had to be given lunch in the car. It took prolonged coaxing to get him out of the car at all. Following this he grew more disturbed and became very overactive, frequently running away, swinging on cupboard doors, and rocking in time to music. When, at the age of 2½, his parents returned to England by boat he refused to go into the nursery with other children. At this time his parents began to think he might be deaf, as he often showed no response to those round him. He was also becoming very frightened of new places and needed security symbols and routines to reassure himself. At bedtime he took seven teddy bears to bed with him, placing three on his left hand and four on his right, and could not go to sleep without this arrangement.

In February 1961, when nearly 4, Roy was referred to a clinic which found no evidence of deafness. In view of this, he was seen by a consultant children's psychiatrist and neurologist who noted that there was no evidence of brain damage and felt this was 'a genuine Kannerian psychosis or infantile autism'. He felt that the child had no real affection for his mother, and noted the gradual accumulation of withdrawal and disinterestedness since the age of 12 months. As an example of his manneristic behaviour, the doctor reported that Roy, when offered sweets, would not eat them until he had sorted them into piles by colour. He suggested that residential treatment would probably eventually be needed.

This need was precipitated in December 1961 when Roy's mother was admitted to hospital with a nervous breakdown. Roy went to a children's home, but was clearly unsuitably placed there, as there were young babies whom he tried to bite and scratch. Some mornings he would refuse to eat anything and then start to scream loudly and continuously. He had an obsession for sweets and biscuits, often refusing to eat anything else. He was generally wet and often soiled as well. Generally he showed little interest but was mesmerized by the vacuum cleaner. He liked to hide behind curtains and stand on window sills, and in more disturbed moments would rip down the curtains, throw toys, and tear books and his own clothes. He was admitted to West Stowell on 22 January 1962, as an emergency.

Roy was then 4½, a well-built child with golden hair and grey eyes. He had recently been tested for phenylketonuria and given an EEG examination, both of which were negative. His mother was still in hospital where she was being treated for depression, but was expected to be out again soon. She had been diagnosed as schizophrenic in a mental hospital a year before, and his grandmother had been in hospital for a time with depression after the menopause. A social worker had described her as a 'plump hysterical little woman'. Roy's father was a tall, thin, unemotional man who said he suffered from migraine headaches. He appeared rather uncertain of himself and his feelings. Roy's parents married young soon after meeting and the marriage seemed reasonably united, although there had always been friction with their families. Father seemed relatively unperturbed about Roy, but mother seemed unable to accept his disability. This led to her becoming upset whenever he was mentioned, and also to remembering him as a perfect baby, almost as if this were a projection of the child she would like to have had.

On admission Roy was unable to talk but seemed to understand what was said, or required of him. He was wet by night, could dress and feed himself, but needed constant supervision, as he was liable to dart off and turn on taps and switches. There was a considerable autistic element in his behaviour, but he seemed more in touch, albeit in a detached way, than many of the children at West Stowell. In undemanding situations he was in fairly good control of his emotions but could erupt if demands were made, or if he were frustrated. In addition to his withdrawal and emotional disturbance, there seemed a strong element of simple retardation. However, he displayed a number of psychotic mannerisms. He was concerned with surfaces, tapping and scratching them. He collected things and obsessionally clung to objects as security symbols. He was placed in a family group and a therapeutic play group, in both of which special efforts were made to develop verbal communication.

Though he was occasionally aggressive towards younger children if provoked, at no stage did Roy's behaviour cause alarm as it had done at the children's home. He settled quite happily into his family group, though at first he would accept nursing and affection only from his housemother. He was resistant to any direct physical control, and disliked having his hair cut or any other form of close attention. He was shyly friendly towards staff, but did not make any spontaneous or positive approach to adults, though often his demeanour seemed to invite affectionate approaches. In his play group he could concentrate enough to do jigsaws and match blocks, but with most toys he was more interested in scratching their surfaces than playing. His play was solitary, and he aggressively resented interference from other children, especially if this was connected with a toy or object he had.

During his first year at West Stowell Roy made no particular progress but maintained the improved level of stability that had been noted on admission. He was a cheerful boy, though solitary and self-centred. He continued to be acquisitive and possessive, and the only times he was aggressive were when another child had a toy he wanted. He resisted relationships except on an infantile basis. When distressed he would sometimes scream with a shrill shriek, but this rarely happened. By the end of his first year in the unit, when he was nearly 6, he seemed a cheerful, lively, outgoing child, operating at a very retarded level, but with some constructive ability. He was clean by day but needed raising at night. Otherwise his behaviour was increasingly conformative and less overactive. He had been home on leave on one or two occasions without any particular trouble, although he continued to show there his previous pattern of attitudes.

By the end of 1963, when nearly 7, Roy was no particular management problem in unstressful situations and seemed to be moving towards the position of a stable subnormal child. His approach to adults seemed essentially for creature comfort, but from time to time he was making his own tentative approaches. Otherwise, there was little basic change in his behaviour. He played almost exclusively alone, was very resistant to change, getting upset even if taken from his play group to another familiar place, and remained possessive of toys and fascinated by surfaces. He would sometimes 'play' at running away or evading authority as if to gain attention.

The above pattern continued throughout 1964. Roy became very attached to a tin box containing burnt matches and was very upset if parted from it. He was also becoming demanding, and would be very upset if there were not an immediate response to his requests. There had been no progress with speech, though his parents said that sometimes at home he would point to a picture book and use words appropriately for pictures in it. His mother had gone into hospital again, and so his visits and leaves were curtailed, but he had taken very well to new houseparents who came in May, and it was hoped this might lead to some advances.

Roy had always been accident-prone as a result of impulsive

behaviour and apparent unawareness of common dangers. In August he broke away from a nurse and dashed in front of a car. He was taken to hospital where he was found to be only superficially injured. As he was very restless and uneasy, wetting and soiling all the time, he was discharged early back to West Stowell. On return he was soon back to his usual state. During the rest of the year he seemed, if anything, to be rather improved. He was less aggressive if frustrated, used a few words, and was rather less preoccupied with surfaces and rattling objects. He also began to develop a shallow relationship with another child, and the two would romp together.

In April 1965 Roy was 8 and had been at West Stowell for over three years. His mother was now out of hospital, but difficulty over leaves continued, as his father had been posted to the Far East. He continued a solitary child, disliking interference from other children, but friendly towards adults.

In the summer Roy was unable to go on holiday, but had a few outings from West Stowell with members of staff while most of the children were away. On one trip he was taken to the seaside, where he spent much of his time in picking up old cartons and other small objects he spied on the beach.

In November 1965 Roy's houseparents left, and this resulted in a temporary regression. He stopped dressing himself, would run away from the table during meals, and temporarily lost toilet control. However, within a month he had returned to his usual behaviour and it was felt that generally he had moved forward over the year. His level of activity was severely limited, but he was showing slightly more interest in his surroundings and seemed less dependent on security symbols, though he still enjoyed shaking a small box in his hands.

At Christmas once again he did not go on leave, but the charge nurse took him into his own family for the holiday period, and reported that Roy was well-behaved and seemed to enjoy himself, especially as there were no other children to compete for attention. He showed great interest in a humming-top given him as a present and used it for the correct purpose. He was toilet-controlled throughout this period.

His behaviour continued to cause no trouble after the holiday, but he was often noticed to be upset by the rather rough and noisy behaviour of other children in his play group, frequently trying to get away to another, quieter group. In view of this he was placed back into the quieter group where he settled happily in an undemanding way, showing no apparent interest in the other children or the play therapist.

In March 1966 Roy was transferred to a more structured group where he settled well. His houseparents thought he had good potential and cited his habit of apparently working out how many plates were needed for each meal, and then putting a cup and plate away if any member of the group was absent. He showed a great fear of being shut in, and would scream if he saw any member of staff locking the door of any room he was in.

In the therapeutic play group Roy was showing an improved capacity for relationships and an interest in sorting shaped objects. In view of this, he was transferred to the formal school class on a part-time basis, for an experimental period. He did very little here, but enjoyed the experience and became very upset when he was not allowed to go back in the afternoon.

By May 1966 Roy was 9 years old. He still did not speak and showed no signs of developing even primitive speech. His obsessional behaviour continued and in many situations he would improvise some form of 'shaking' equipment. This might be a piece of paper and some beads, or a large cardboard box and lumps of rock. He would spend hours shaking such objects, unless distracted by staff. He also liked to be chased, and would provoke staff into doing this. If taken for walks, he had to be held tightly, as he still tended to dart off impulsively, regardless of traffic. If upset or frustrated, his initial reaction was often to bite his wrist, and if the frustration was extreme, as in being brought in from the gardens before he was ready, he sometimes went beyond this, screaming and hitting his face violently and making his nose bleed. His parents were still abroad and so could not visit him, which meant that he had no leaves or visits. Roy did not appear aware of this, but it was felt that his future progress would be dependent on his parents eventually being able to play a larger part in his life, which they had always said they hoped to do. Although his progress was slow, there seemed reason to hope that Roy would eventually be able to live outside hospital in a protected environment.

P

References

BENDER, L. (1947). 'Childhood Schizophrenia; a clinical survey of 100 cases', *American Journal of Orthopsychiatry*, **17**, 40–56.

BETTELHEIM, B. (1950). *Love is not Enough*. Glencoe, Ill.: The Free Press.

— (1955 *Truants from Life*. New York: Collier-Macmillan.

CREAK, E. M. *et al* (1961a). 'Schizophrenic Syndrome in Childhood', *British Medical Journal*, **2**, 431.

—— (1961b) 'Schizophrenic Syndrome in Children', *Lancet*, **ii**, 818.

DESPERT, J. L. (1958). 'Further Examination of Diagnostic Criteria in Schizophrenic Illness and Psychoses of Childhood', *American Journal of Psychiatry*, **114**, 784.

GELLNER, L. (1957). 'Some Contemplations about the Border Country between "Mental Deficiency" and Childhood Schizophrenia.'
Paper read to 2nd International Congress for Psychiatry.

—— (1969). A Neurophysiological Concept of Mental Retardation and its Educational Implications. The Dr J. D. Levinson Res. Foundation for Mentally Retarded Children, Chicago.

GILLIES, S. (1965). 'Some Abilities of Psychotic Children and Subnormal Controls', *Journal of Mental Deficiency Research*, **9**, 89.

GILLIES, S., MITTLER, P. and SIMON, B. (1963). 'Some Characteristics of a Group of Psychotic Children and their Families'. Paper to British Psychological Society conference in Reading.

GOLD, S., and SELLER, M. J. (1965). 'An Epileptic Factor in the Serum of Psychotic Children', *Medical Journal of Australia*, **2**, 876.

GOLDFARB, W. (1961). *Childhood Schizophrenia*. Cambridge, Mass.: Harvard University Press.

HERMELIN, B., and O'CONNOR, N. (1964). 'Effects of Sensory Input and Sensory Dominance on severely disturbed Autistic Children and on Subnormal Controls', *British Journal of Psychiatry*, **5**, 201–206.

—— 'Visual Imperception in Psychotic Children', *British Journal of Psychology*, **56**, 453–460.

KAHAN, V. L. (1963). 'The Treatment of Severely Disturbed Children', *Lancet*, February, 319–321.

KANNER, L. (1955). *Child Psychiatry* (4th Edition). Oxford: Black-well.

LAING, R. D., and ESTERSON, A. (1964). *Sanity, Madness, and the Family*. London: Tavistock.

MAIR, K. J. (1963). 'The Behaviour and Abilities of some Psychotic Patients'. Unpublished research report.

O'CONNOR, N. and HERMELIN, B. (1963). 'Measures of Distance and Motility in Psychotic Children and Severely Subnormal Controls', *British Journal of Social and Clinical Psychology*, 3, 29–33.

RIMLAND, B. (1964). *Infantile Autism*. New York: Appleton Century Crofts.

RUTTER, M. (1965). 'The Influence of Organic and Emotional Factors on the Origins, Nature and Outcome of Childhood Psychosis', *Developmental Medicine & Child Neurology* 7, 518.

—— (1966). 'Behavioural and Cognitive Characteristics of a series of Psychotic Children', (to be published in *Childhood Autism* (ed.) J. Wing. London: (Pergamon).

SCHAIN, R. J., and YANNET, H. (1960). 'Infantile Autism. An analysis of 50 cases and a consideration of certain relevant neuro-physiological concepts', *Journal of Pediatrics*, 57, 560.

SIMON, G. B., and GILLIES, S. M. (1964). 'Some Physical Characteristics of a Group of Psychotic Children', *British Journal of Psychiat.*, 110, 464.

TIZARD, J. (1960). 'Residential Care of Mentally Handicapped Children', *British Medical Journal*, i, 1041–1046.

WING, L. (1964). *Autistic Children*. National Association for Mentally Handicapped Children.

Index

abnormal behaviour
  distinct from maladjustment, xi-xii
  and recognition of psychosis, 48–9,
    125–6, 136, 183
Ackerman, P. R., and autism, 8
acting out, xiv, xv, xvii
  in conduct disorders, 82
  of parental attitudes, 53
  psychotherapeutic treatment, 83
adopted children, 51, 105
adrenalin, lessening output, 11–12
affection, response to, xviii, 178–9, 180
aggressiveness, 17
  form of conduct disorder, xviii, 82
  in discharged patients, 93
  inward-turning, xviii
  occurrence in groups, 19, 26–7
  removal in play groups, 76
  response to normality, 81
  towards other children, 146, 151,
    157, 162–6 *passim*, 177, 192, 198–
    202 *passim*
  parents, 148–9
  staff, 147, 151, 154, 164
anger, negative transference, 83
antisocial behaviour
  after hospitalization, 52
  and mental illness, xv, xviii
  during psychotherapy, 83
aphasia, 129, 131, 141
asphyxia, 42, 43, 59, 168
attacks on other children
  group reaction, 65
  by psychotic-severely subnormal, 17
  in case histories, 126, 136, 146, 147
autism, xiv, xvii
  age of onset, 46, 48
  approach to, 6
  arrested emotional development, 60
  'early infantile', 46
  level of intelligence, 7
  interest in, xv, 7
  pattern of mental illness, xvi
  'Nine Points', 9
  and organic causes, 8, 133

parental responsibility, 7–8
perceptual difficulties, 8
failure in primary relationships, 11
differentiated from psychosis, 15
compared with 'psychotic' and
  'juvenile schizophrenia', 16
resistance to change, 7, 14
scientific observations, 7
and self-punishment, xviii
precipitated by stress, 13
symptoms (infantile and childhood),
  7, 12–13, 46
response to treatment, xvii
autistic children, 15, 17
  appearance and intelligence, 67
  and 'heightened experiences', 71
  inaccessibility, 19–20
  indifference to adults, 19
  manneristic activities, 32, 67–8
  in play groups, 75
  and psychotherapy, 84, 96
  sensory abnormalities, 25
  social class of parents, 56, 98
  speech abnormalities, 24–5, 68, 84,
    96, 182
  toilet patterns, 25
  response to treatment, 95
  case histories, 67–8, 84, 105, 111,
    112–13, 116, 129–34, 182–6, 188,
    199–205

balletic movements, xiii
  occurrence in groups, 20–1
bed-stripping, 27, 64–5
  in case histories, 145, 147, 151, 152
bed-wetting, 146
  aids to improvement, 64
  in case histories, 152–3, 178–9
  see also enuresis
Bender, Lauretta
  and 'childhood schizophrenia', 8
  'pseudoneurotic syndrome', 17
Bettelheim, B.,
  and autism, 8
  and parental participation, 86

209

Index

Bettelheim, B. *contd*
and Sonia Shankman Orthogenic School, 10
birth trauma, 38
four categories, 42–4
frequency and severity, 40, 42
in groups studied, 39, 42–4
information studied, 40–1
in case histories, 105, 112, 140, 162, 168, 176, 182, 200
biting, 27
blindness, 40, 95
Bowlby, J., and maternal deprivation, 52
brain abnormality
part in development, xv
investigations into, 38 ff.
brain damage, xv
distinguished from autism, 7
in discharged patients, 95
and emotional deprivation, xiii
evidence looked for, 38, 39
eye movements, 36
and mental illness, xi
and motor abnormalities, 20
and organic schizophrenia, 8
in subnormality, 13, 58
in case histories, 111, 113, 131, 141, 178
brain dysfunction, and psychosis, 37
brain infection, 43
brain investigations
retarded bone-age, 13, 38, 39–40
indication of organic condition, 44
unrelated to poor prognosis, 45
EEG, 13, 38, 39, 40, 95
skull X-ray, 13, 39
breast-feeding, part-object relationship, xi

central nervous system
abnormalities, 156
organic immaturity, 8
cerebral palsy, 39
chaotic personality disturbance, xiv, xvi, xvii
response to treatment, xvii
child-centred intensive care, xiii, 60 ff.
adult behaviour, 61
and emotional deprivation, 96
and individuality, 62
treatment of group reactions, 65–6

method of approach, 6, 14, 61
and misbehaviour, 66
absence of punishment, 66
purpose of, xiii, xiv, 60
and reactive conduct disorders, 69
setting demanded, 14, 61
effect of staff changes, 69–70
special events, 71–2, 115, 159, 160
in case histories, 105, 111, 117, 129, 135, 140, 145, 161, 168, 176, 190 200
child guidance services, xi–xii, 130, 162, 163
child management, 56, 160
varying patterns, 53, 54
children's homes
patients from, 156, 158, 161, 162, 163–7 *passim*, 199
climbing, motor abnormality, 21
in case histories, 117, 118, 143, 144, 189, 194
clothes-tearing, 27
use in tranquillizers, 80
in case histories, 68, 148, 152, 153, 161
clumsiness, motor abnormality, 20
coloured children, 162
aggression in, 67
sensitivity, 165–6
Conduct Disorders (diagnostic category), xii, xvii, 16
abnormal infantile behaviour, 48–50
accompanying disturbances, xvii
aetiology, 12
age of onset and recognition, 48
aggressive and destructive behaviour, 26–7
anxiety-ridden, 14
birth data, 40, 41, 42, 44, 59, 162, 176
bone-age, 44, 45
brain damage, 38, 39
childish rather than pathological, xiii–xiv
diagnosis and prognosis, 17, 79, 90, 91, 97
family background, 59
miscellaneous symptoms, 36–7
motor abnormalities, 21
obsessional behaviour, 29
organic defects, 40
parental involvement, 38, 54, 55, 56, 57, 58, 60

210

psychic trauma, 50–1
psychotherapy and, 82, 84
reactive elements, 58
referral pattern, 57
self-punishment, 28
sensory experiences, 26
social class, 56, 57
speech abnormalities, 24, 49
toilet patterns, 23
response to treatment, xvii, 91, 96,
    104
vulnerability, 38
case histories, 18, 19, 67, 161–7,
    176–82
congenital disorders, 39, 43, 44
convulsions, 39, 40, 112, 176
cranial trauma, in subnormality, 13
Creak, E. M.,
'Nine Points' of childhood schizo-
    phrenia, 9–10, 15, 25, 97
cretinism, 39, 95

day nurseries, 191, 192
deafness
communication with, 67, 179–81
in case histories, 67, 179–81
deafness (apparent), 25
in case histories, 121, 129, 130–1,
    140, 143, 154, 155, 156, 201
death, obsession with, 123–6 *passim*,
    148
depression, parental, 58, 167, 170, 202
Despert, J. L., 53
and autism, 7–8
destructiveness, 15
in groups studied, 20, 26–7, 34
negative transference, 83
in case histories, 116, 117, 120, 145,
    147, 199, 201
Disturbed Subnormal (diagnostic cate-
    gory), xiv, 16, 17
abnormal infantile behaviour, 48–50
age of onset and recognition, 48
aggressive and destructive be-
    haviour, 26–7
birth data, 40, 41, 42, 44
bone-age, 44, 45
post-discharge history, 92–3, 94, 95
miscellaneous symptoms, 36–7
motor abnormalities, 20, 21
obsessional behaviour, 29
organic defects, 39, 40

parents' mental state, 55, 56, 58
in play groups, 75
prognosis, 17, 90, 91
psychic trauma, 50–1
response to psychotherapy, 84
response to treatment, 91, 96, 104
self-punishment, 28
sensory experiences, 26
social class, 56, 57
speech abnormalities, 24
drawings, reflection of fantasies, 163
drug-free observation, xiii, 80–1
drug therapy, 134, 137–8, 185, 198

ear-eye covering, 25
echolalia, 23, 24
in play groups, 76
during psychotherapy, 83
in case histories, 109, 137, 170, 193–4,
    195
educational subnormality
school provision, 78, 79, 93, 109,
    124, 156, 167
Eisenberg, L., and autism, 7–8
emotional abnormality, xii, xvii
emotional deprivation
acting-out children, xiv
approach to, 6
varying effects, xv
and psychotic children, 58
emotional disturbances
and birth trauma, 43
broad symptoms, 17
parental, 55, 56
and toilet control, 22
in case histories, 129, 141
emotional immaturity, 161, 163
emotional instability
and childhood immaturity, xv
parental, 98, 142, 155, 183
micro-psychic trauma, 50
in case histories, 126, 170, 202
encephalitis, 58
encopresis
in groups studied, 22, 23, 27
play therapists and, 75–6
use of tranquillizers, 80
treatment, 64
in case histories, 67, 68, 153, 177,
    186, 195, 201
enuresis
in groups studied, 22, 23, 25, 36